T0383244

New Directions in Behavioral Intervention Development for Pediatric Obesity

Editor

SYLVIE NAAR

PEDIATRIC CLINICS OF NORTH AMERICA

www.pediatric.theclinics.com

Consulting Editor
BONITA F. STANTON

June 2016 • Volume 63 • Number 3

ELSEVIER

1600 John F. Kennedy Boulevard • Suite 1800 • Philadelphia, Pennsylvania, 19103-2899

http://www.theclinics.com

THE PEDIATRIC CLINICS OF NORTH AMERICA Volume 63, Number 3
June 2016 ISSN 0031-3955, ISBN-13: 978-0-323-44626-6

Editor: Kerry Holland
Developmental Editor: Casey Jackson

The Pediatric Clinics of North America (ISSN 0031-3955) is published bimonthly by Elsevier Inc., 360 Park Avenue South, New York, NY 10010-1710. Months of issue are February, April, June, August, October, and December. Periodicals postage paid at New York, NY and additional mailing offices. Subscription prices are $200.00 per year (US individuals), $556.00 per year (US institutions), $270.00 per year (Canadian individuals), $740.00 per year (Canadian institutions), $325.00 per year (international individuals), $740.00 per year (international institutions), $100.00 per year (US students and residents), and $165.00 per year (international and Canadian residents and students). To receive students/resident rare, orders must be accompanied by name of affiliated institution, date of term, and the signature of program/residency coordinator on institution letterhead. Orders will be billed at individual rate until proof of status is received. Foreign air speed delivery is included in all *Clinics* subscription prices. All prices are subject to change without notice. **POSTMASTER:** Send address changes to *The Pediatric Clinics of North America*, Elsevier Health Sciences Division, Subscription Customer Service, 3251 Riverport Lane, Maryland Heights, MO 63043. **Customer Service: 1-800-654-2452 (US and Canada). From outside of the US and Canada: 1-314-447-8871. Fax: 1-314-447-8029. For print support, E-mail: JournalsCustomerService-usa@elsevier.com. For online support, E-mail: JournalsOnlineSupport-usa@elsevier.com.**

Reprints. For copies of 100 or more, of articles in this publication, please contact the Commercial Reprints Department, Elsevier Inc., 360 Park Avenue South, New York, NY 10010-1710. Tel.: 212-633-3874; Fax: 212-633-3820; E-mail: reprints@elsevier.com.

The Pediatric Clinics of North America is also published in Spanish by McGraw-Hill Inter-americana Editores S.A., Mexico City, Mexico; in Portuguese by Riechmann and Affonso Editores, Rua Comandante Coelho 1085, CEP 21250, Rio de Janeiro, Brazil; and in Greek by Althayia SA, Athens, Greece.

The Pediatric Clinics of North America is covered in *MEDLINE/PubMed (Index Medicus), Excerpta Medica, Current Contents, Current Contents/Clinical Medicine, Science Citation Index, ASCA, ISI/BIOMED,* and *BIOSIS.*

PROGRAM OBJECTIVE

The goal of the *Pediatric Clinics of North America* is to keep practicing physicians and residents up to date with current clinical practice in pediatrics by providing timely articles reviewing the state-of-the-art in patient care.

TARGET AUDIENCE

All practicing pediatricians, physicians and healthcare professionals who provide patient care to pediatric patients.

LEARNING OBJECTIVES

Upon completion of this activity, participants will be able to:
1. Review neurocognitive processes and interventions in pediatric obesity.
2. Discuss behavioral economic factors and stress-obesity research in pediatrics.
3. Recognize strategies in basic behavioural science and behavioural sleep integration as approaches for pediatric children.

ACCREDITATION

The Elsevier Office of Continuing Medical Education (EOCME) is accredited by the Accreditation Council for Continuing Medical Education (ACCME) to provide continuing medical education for physicians.

The EOCME designates this enduring material for a maximum of 15 *AMA PRA Category 1 Credit*(s)™. Physicians should claim only the credit commensurate with the extent of their participation in the activity.

All other health care professionals requesting continuing education credit for this enduring material will be issued a certificate of participation.

DISCLOSURE OF CONFLICTS OF INTEREST

The EOCME assesses conflict of interest with its instructors, faculty, planners, and other individuals who are in a position to control the content of CME activities. All relevant conflicts of interest that are identified are thoroughly vetted by EOCME for fair balance, scientific objectivity, and patient care recommendations. EOCME is committed to providing its learners with CME activities that promote improvements or quality in healthcare and not a specific proprietary business or a commercial interest.

The planning committee, staff, authors and editors listed below have identified no financial relationships or relationships to products or devices they or their spouse/life partner have with commercial interest related to the content of this CME activity:

Terrance Albrecht, PhD; Kathryn E. Brogan Hartlieb, PhD, RD; Eduardo E. Bustamante, PhD; April Carcone, PhD; Lisa M. Clifford, PhD; Susan M. Czajkowski, PhD; Catherine L. Davis, PhD, FTOS; Amy J. Fahrenkamp, MA; Anjali Fortna; Mark K. Greenwald, PhD; Donna Harris, MA; Chantelle N. Hart, PhD; Nicola L. Hawley, PhD; Kerry Holland; Angela J. Jacques-Tiura, PhD; Indu Kumari; Tim Martin, PhD; Mary Beth McCullough, PhD; Rada Mihalcea, PhD; Alison L. Miller, PhD; Sylvie Naar, PhD; Veronica Perez-Rosas, PhD; Ken Resnicow, PhD; Amy F. Sato, PhD; Robert P. Schwartz, MD; Linda Snetselaar, PhD, RD, FAND; Bonita F. Stanton, MD; Lori J. Stark, PhD; Cathleen Odar Stough, PhD; Megan Suermann; Elizabeth K. Towner, PhD; Richard Wasserman, MD, MPH; Celestine F. Williams, MS; Rena R. Wing, PhD.

UNAPPROVED/OFF-LABEL USE DISCLOSURE

The EOCME requires CME faculty to disclose to the participants:
1. When products or procedures being discussed are off-label, unlabelled, experimental, and/or investigational (not US Food and Drug Administration [FDA] approved); and
2. Any limitations on the information presented, such as data that are preliminary or that represent ongoing research, interim analyses, and/or unsupported opinions. Faculty may discuss information about pharmaceutical agents that is outside of FDA-approved labelling. This information is intended solely for CME and is not intended to promote off-label use of these medications. If you have any questions, contact the medical affairs department of the manufacturer for the most recent prescribing information.

TO ENROLL

To enroll in the *Pediatric Clinics of North America* Continuing Medical Education program, call customer service at 1-800-654-2452 or sign up online at http://www.theclinics.com/home/cme. The CME program is available to subscribers for an additional annual fee of USD 290.

METHOD OF PARTICIPATION

In order to claim credit, participants must complete the following:

1. Complete enrolment as indicated above.
2. Read the activity.
3. Complete the CME Test and Evaluation. Participants must achieve a score of 70% on the test. All CME Tests and Evaluations must be completed online.

CME INQUIRIES/SPECIAL NEEDS

For all CME inquiries or special needs, please contact elsevierCME@elsevier.com.

Contributors

CONSULTING EDITOR

BONITA F. STANTON, MD
Founding Dean and Professor of Pediatrics, Seton Hall University-Hackensack-Meridian School of Medicine; President, Academic Enterprise, Hackensack University Health Network South Orange, New Jersey

EDITOR

SYLVIE NAAR, PhD
Professor and Director, Division of Behavioral Sciences, Department of Family Medicine and Public Health Sciences, Wayne State School of Medicine, Integrative Biosciences Center, Detroit, Michigan

AUTHORS

TERRANCE ALBRECHT, PhD
Department of Oncology, Wayne State University-Karmanos Cancer Institute, Detroit, Michigan

KATHRYN E. BROGAN HARTLIEB, PhD, RD
Department of Dietetics and Nutrition, Robert Stempel College of Public Health and Social Work, Florida International University, Miami, Florida

EDUARDO E. BUSTAMANTE, PhD
Assistant Professor, Department of Kinesiology and Nutrition, College of Applied Health Sciences, University of Illinois at Chicago, Chicago, Illinois

APRIL IDALSKI CARCONE, PhD
Department of Family Medicine and Public Health Sciences, Wayne State University School of Medicine, Detroit, Michigan

LISA M. CLIFFORD, PhD
Research Assistant Professor, Department of Clinical and Health Psychology, College of Public Health and Health Professions, University of Florida, Gainesville, Florida

SUSAN M. CZAJKOWSKI, PhD
Chief, Health Behaviors Research Branch, Behavioral Research Program, Division of Cancer Control and Population Sciences, National Cancer Institute, National Institutes of Health, Rockville, Maryland

CATHERINE L. DAVIS, PhD, FTOS
Professor, Pediatrics, Georgia Prevention Institute, Medical College of Georgia, Augusta University, Augusta, Georgia

AMY J. FAHRENKAMP, MA
Graduate Research Assistant, Department of Psychological Sciences, Kent State University, Kent, Ohio

MARK K. GREENWALD, PhD
Professor, Department of Psychiatry and Behavioral Neurosciences, School of Medicine; Department of Pharmacy Practice, Eugene Applebaum College of Pharmacy and Health Sciences, iBio –Behavioral Health, Wayne State University, Detroit, Michigan

DONNA HARRIS, MA
Research Associate, Pediatric Research in Office Settings (PROS), Department of Research, American Academy of Pediatrics, Elk Grove Village, Illinois

CHANTELLE N. HART, PhD
Associate Professor, Department of Social and Behavioral Sciences, Center for Obesity Research and Education, College of Public Health, Temple University, Philadelphia, Pennsylvania

NICOLA L. HAWLEY, PhD
Assistant Professor, Department of Chronic Disease Epidemiology, Yale School of Public Health, New Haven, Connecticut

ANGELA J. JACQUES-TIURA, PhD
Assistant Professor, Department of Family Medicine and Public Health Sciences, School of Medicine, iBio – Behavioral Health, Wayne State University, Detroit, Michigan

TIM MARTIN, PhD
Department of Psychology, Kennesaw State University, Kennesaw, Georgia

MARY BETH McCULLOUGH, PhD
Post-Doctoral Research Fellow, Division of Behavioral Medicine and Clinical Psychology, Cincinnati Children's Hospital Medical Center, Cincinnati, Ohio

RADA MIHALCEA, PhD
Professor, Department of Electrical Engineering and Computer Science, University of Michigan, Ann Arbor, Michigan

ALISON L. MILLER, PhD
Associate Professor, Department of Health Behavior and Health Education, University of Michigan School of Public Health, Center for Human Growth and Development, Ann Arbor, Michigan

VERONICA PEREZ-ROSAS, PhD
Post Doctoral Student, Department of Electrical Engineering and Computer Science, University of Michigan, Ann Arbor, Michigan

KEN RESNICOW, PhD
Professor, Department of Health Behavior and Health Education, School of Public Health, University of Michigan, Ann Arbor, Michigan

AMY F. SATO, PhD
Assistant Professor, Department of Psychological Sciences, Kent State University, Kent, Ohio

ROBERT P. SCHWARTZ, MD
Professor Emeritus, Office of Emeritus Affairs, Wake Forest School of Medicine, Winston-Salem, North Carolina

LINDA SNETSELAAR, PhD, RD, FAND
Department of Epidemiology, College of Public Health, University of Iowa, Iowa City, Iowa

LORI J. STARK, PhD
Professor, Division of Behavioral Medicine and Clinical Psychology, Cincinnati Children's Hospital Medical Center, Cincinnati, Ohio

CATHLEEN ODAR STOUGH, PhD
Post-Doctoral Research Fellow, Division of Behavioral Medicine and Clinical Psychology, Cincinnati Children's Hospital Medical Center, Cincinnati, Ohio

ELIZABETH K. TOWNER, PhD
Assistant Professor, Department of Family Medicine and Public Health Sciences, Wayne State University School of Medicine, Wayne State University, Detroit, Michigan

RICHARD WASSERMAN, MD, MPH
Department of Pediatrics, University of Vermont College of Medicine, Burlington, Vermont; Pediatric Research in Office Settings, American Academy of Pediatrics, Elk Grove Village, Illinois

CELESTINE F. WILLIAMS, MS
Research Associate, Georgia Prevention Institute, Augusta University, Augusta, Georgia

RENA R. WING, PhD
Professor, Department of Psychiatry and Human Behavior, Weight Control and Diabetes Research Center, The Miriam Hospital, Alpert Medical School of Brown University, Providence, Rhode Island

Contents

National Institutes of Health Update: Translating Basic Behavioral Science into New Pediatric Obesity Interventions

Susan M. Czajkowski

Pediatric obesity increases the risk of later-life obesity and chronic diseases. Basic research to better understand factors associated with excessive weight gain in early life and studies translating research findings into preventive and therapeutic strategies are essential to our ability to better prevent and treat childhood obesity. This overview describes several National Institutes of Health efforts designed to stimulate basic and translational research in childhood obesity prevention and treatment. These examples demonstrate the value of research in early phase translational pediatric obesity research and highlight some promising directions for this important area of research.

From Bench to Bedside: Understanding Stress-Obesity Research Within the Context of Translation to Improve Pediatric Behavioral Weight Management

Amy F. Sato and Amy J. Fahrenkamp

A growing body of literature suggests that stress, including chronic stress and acute physiologic stress reactivity, is one contributor to the development and maintenance of obesity in youth. Little has been done to apply the literature on stress and obesity risk to inform the development of pediatric behavioral weight control (BWC) interventions. The aims of this review are to (1) discuss research linking stress and pediatric obesity, (2) provide examples of the implications of the stress-obesity research for pediatric BWC development, and (3) propose that a mindfulness-based approach may be useful in targeting stress reduction within pediatric BWC.

Behavioral Economic Factors Related to Pediatric Obesity

Angela J. Jacques-Tiura and Mark K. Greenwald

Behavioral economics (BE) suggests that food and activity choices are governed by costs, available alternatives, and reinforcement. This article reviews basic, translational, and intervention research using a BE framework with overweight or obese children up to age 18. We address BE concepts and methods, and discuss developmental issues, the continuum of

BE intervention approaches, findings of studies focused on increasing the cost of unwanted behaviors (ie, energy-dense food intake and sedentary behavior) and decreasing the cost of desired behaviors (ie, healthy food intake and PA), and our team's recent basic behavioral studies using BE approaches with minority adolescents.

Childhood obesily is a significant problem in the United States, but current childhood obesity prevention approaches have limited efficacy. Self-regulation processes organize behavior to achieve a goal and may shape health behaviors and health outcomes. Obesity prevention approaches that focus on the cognitive and behavioral mechanisms that underlie self-regulation early in life may therefore lead to better outcomes. This article reviews the development of executive functioning (EF), identifies influences on EF development, discusses aspects of EF relating to increased risk for childhood obesity, and considers how EF-weight associations may change across development. Implications for intervention are discussed.

This article examines cognitive, academic, and brain outcomes of physical activity in overweight or obese youth, with attention to minority youth who experience health disparities. Physically active academic lessons may have greater immediate cognitive and academic benefits among overweight and obese children than normal-weight children. Quasi-experimental studies testing physical activity programs in overweight and obese youth show promise; a few randomized controlled trials including African Americans show efficacy. Thus, making academic lessons physically active may improve inhibition and attentiveness, particularly in overweight youngsters. Regular physical activity may be efficacious for improving neurologic, cognitive, and achievement outcomes in overweight or obese youth.

Developing interventions targeting obesity reduction in preschoolers is an emergent area. Although intensive, multicomponent interventions seem a promising approach to preschool obesity reduction, this review identifies and discusses approaches to 3 critical gaps (poor reach to families from low-income and minority backgrounds, lack of sufficient evidence to determine the most effective and efficient treatment components and approaches to treating obesity in early childhood, and lack of consensus on how best to discern intervention effectiveness) that need to be addressed to advance the preschool obesity literature.

Despite being the focus of widespread public health efforts, childhood obesity remains an epidemic worldwide. Given the now well-documented consequences of obesity for childhood health and psychosocial functioning, as well as associated morbidity in adulthood, identifying novel, modifiable behaviors that can be targeted to improve weight control is imperative. Enhancing children's sleep may show promise in assisting with weight regulation. The present paper describes the development of a brief behavioral sleep intervention for school-aged children, including preliminary findings of this work as well as areas for future study.

Effective patient–provider communication is not a primary focus of medical school curricula. Motivational interviewing (MI) is a patient-centered, directive communication framework appropriate for in health care. Research on MI's causal mechanisms has established patient change talk as a mediator of behavior change. Current MI research focuses on identifying which provider communication skills are responsible for evoking change talk. MI recommends informing, asking, and listening. Research provides evidence that asking for and reflecting patient change talk are effective communication strategies, but cautions providers to inform judiciously. Supporting a patient's decision making autonomy is an important strategy to promote health behaviors.

Rates of childhood obesity in the United States remain at historic highs. The pediatric primary care office represents an important yet underused setting to intervene with families. One factor contributing to underuse of the primary care setting is lack of effective available interventions. One evidence-based method to help engage and motivate patients is motivational interviewing, a client-centered and goal-oriented style of counseling used extensively to increase autonomous motivation and modify health behaviors. This article summarizes the methods and results from a large trial implemented in primary care pediatric office and concludes with recommendations for improving the intervention and increasing its dissemination.

PEDIATRIC CLINICS OF NORTH AMERICA

Foreword

New Directions in Behavioral Intervention Development for Pediatric Obesity

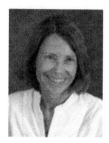

Bonita F. Stanton, MD
Consulting Editor

Since the appearance of Homo sapiens some 200,000 years ago, a primary challenge to mankind has been finding, acquiring, and consuming sufficient food sources to meet current and future metabolic needs. These internal energy sources must be readily available to meet metabolic demands, but are also carefully guarded by the body to sustain life over lean periods. The body developed exquisite and redundant mechanisms to protect this life-sustaining energy system over many scores of thousands of years.

And then, beginning in the twentieth century, the whole paradigm on which this exquisite system was based changed. For most citizens in industrialized nations and a large proportion of those in emerging and nonindustrialized nations, calories have become too abundant. Rather than needing mechanisms to protect and enhance internal food storage, our bodies are faced with an inability to expend a sufficient proportion of consumed calories. Without sufficient time to adapt, our bodies continue to follow the only script that they have—the script that they have mastered over the millennia to preserve at great effort these calories. And thus, the epidemic of obesity was born and is flourishing.

Certainly there is no easy answer to this problem. The more we learn about the cause of obesity and the body's responses, the less sanguine we become about simple dieting measures and/or medicinal approaches as being sufficient to address the problem.

The articles in this issue are very important for practicing pediatricians. The articles provide a solid background to understand the complexities involved in preventing and treating obesity and a wide array of approaches that are available. Moreover, they provide detailed descriptions of programmatic approaches to working with children and families who are impacted and/or may be impacted. This issue enables the practitioner to move far beyond simply recommending dieting and empowers him or her to be an

Pediatr Clin N Am 63 (2016) xiii–xiv
http://dx.doi.org/10.1016/j.pcl.2016.03.003
0031-3955/16/$ – see front matter © 2016 Published by Elsevier Inc.

active, informed partner in supporting and guiding a child's and family's campaign to overcome and/or avoid obesity.

Bonita F. Stanton, MD
School of Medicine
Seton Hall University
400 South Orange Avenue
South Orange, NJ 07079, USA

E-mail address:
bonita.stanton@shu.edu

Preface

From Bench to Bedside: T1 Translation of Basic Behavioral Science into Novel Pediatric Obesity Interventions

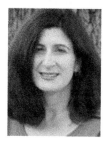

Sylvie Naar, PhD
Editor

As 40% of premature deaths can be attributed to preventable behavioral factors, the single greatest opportunity to improve health lies in changing personal behavior such as diet and physical activity.[1,2] Yet, one out of every three US children is overweight or obese, and obesity rates have not declined among minority youth.[3] There are many reasons for this lack of progress in incorporating successful healthy lifestyle treatments into pediatric care and community settings, and one critical concern involves the limited "pool" of efficacious behavioral treatments available. There are limited efficacious pediatric obesity interventions available for clinical and community settings,[4] and successful weight loss trials for minority youth are rare.[5] Even fewer interventions have been shown to significantly improve clinical health outcomes such as adiposity, glucose intolerance, blood pressure, and cholesterol level,[6] and maintenance of behavior change over the long term remains a challenge.

According to the Institute of Medicine, the first stage of translational research (T1) focuses on "the transfer of new understandings of disease mechanisms gained in the laboratory into the development of new methods for diagnosis, therapy, and prevention and their first testing in humans."[7] T1 research in which "bench" findings are applied to the "bedside" is less common in the behavioral arena. Thus, advances in our understanding of fundamental human processes, such as motivation, emotion, cognition, self-regulation, communication, stress, and social networks, are not being optimally applied to our most pressing behavioral health problems. This issue focuses on promising behavioral treatments for pediatric obesity "in the pipeline" that have been translated from basic behavioral science and are the process of refinement and proof of concept testing. In this issue, Czajkowski and colleagues describe the

Pediatr Clin N Am 63 (2016) xv–xvi
http://dx.doi.org/10.1016/j.pcl.2016.03.002
0031-3955/16/$ – see front matter © 2016 Published by Elsevier Inc.

pediatric.theclinics.com

ORBIT model for behavioral intervention development, and the first eight articles in this issue describe studies that address designing and preliminary testing of new interventions per the ORBIT model. The last article (Resnicow and colleagues) describes new directions in the implementation of an evidence-based practice in primary care settings. We thank the authors for their commitment to the dissemination of promising strategies to curb the obesity epidemic.

Sylvie Naar, PhD
Department of Family Medicine
and Public Health Sciences
Wayne State School of Medicine
Integrative Biosciences Center
Behavioral Health (H206)
6135 Woodward Avenue
Detroit, MI 48202, USA

E-mail address:
snaarkin@med.wayne.edu

REFERENCES

1. Schroeder SA. We can do better—improving the health of the American people. N Engl J Med 2007;357(12):1221–8.
2. National Institute of Health. Office of behavioral and social science research: behavior change and maintenance. 2012. Available at: https://obssrarchive.od.nih.gov/scientific_areas/health_behaviour/behaviour_changes/index.aspx. Accessed January 18, 2012.
3. Ogden CL, Carroll MD, Kit BK, et al. Prevalence of childhood and adult obesity in the United States, 2011-2012. JAMA 2014;311(8):806–14.
4. Janicke DM, Steele RG, Gayes LA, et al. Systematic review and meta-analysis of comprehensive behavioral family lifestyle interventions addressing pediatric obesity. J Pediatr Psychol 2014;39(8):809–25.
5. Wilson DK. New perspectives on health disparities and obesity interventions in youth. J Pediatr Psychol 2009;34(3):231–44.
6. Peirson L, Fitzpatrick-Lewis D, Morrison K, et al. Treatment of overweight and obesity in children and youth: a systematic review and meta-analysis. CMAJ Open 2015;3(1):E35–46.
7. Sung NS, Crowley WF Jr, Genel M, et al. Central challenges facing the national clinical research enterprise. JAMA 2003;289(10):1278–87.

Errata

Please note the following corrections: In the October 2013 issue of *Pediatric Clinics of North America* (Volume 60, Issue 5) in the list of contributors (page 5) and in the article, "Common Office Procedures and Analgesia Considerations" (page 163): The author's name originally appeared as Amy Baxter (Baxter, A) and should be changed to Amy L. Baxter (Baxter, AL).

In the April 2016 issue (Volume 63, Issue 2) of *Pediatric Clinics* Mark Arbore, BSN, RN, CPN is the co-author of "Measurement, Standards, and Peer Benchmarking: One Hospital's Journey," with Brian S. Martin, DMD, MHCDS.

In the December 2014 (Volume 61, Issue 6) issue of Pediatric Clinics, the video accompanying the article "Assessment and Treatment of Hip Pain in the Adolescent Athlete" by Brian D. Giordano, MD on Pages 1137–1154 has been removed, as it was published in error.

Pediatr Clin N Am 63 (2016) xvii
http://dx.doi.org/10.1016/j.pcl.2016.03.001
0031-3955/16/$ – see front matter © 2016 Elsevier Inc. All rights reserved.

pediatric.theclinics.com

National Institutes of Health Update: Translating Basic Behavioral Science into New Pediatric Obesity Interventions

CrossMark

Susan M. Czajkowski, PhD

KEYWORDS

- Basic behavioral science • Early phase behavioral translation
- Intervention development • Pediatric obesity
- Obesity-related behavioral intervention trials (ORBIT) model

KEY POINTS

- Pediatric obesity is a common and important risk factor for future obesity and for chronic diseases.
- Basic behavioral research and early phase trials that translate knowledge into interventions to prevent or reduce obesity are important.
- The National Institutes of Health (NIH) supports basic and early phase translational behavioral research related to pediatric obesity through a variety of mechanisms.
- Findings from NIH-supported research in basic and early phase translational behavioral science are producing new discoveries that can be used to develop novel targets for pediatric obesity interventions.
- NIH support is critical to ensure progress in developing, testing, and ultimately implementing new and more effective interventions to reduce pediatric obesity.

INTRODUCTION

Excessive, early weight gain has been found to increase risk for obesity later in life,[1,2] and is a risk factor for many diseases, such as cancer, cardiovascular disease, and diabetes.[3,4] Pediatric obesity has been increasing steadily over the past 3 decades and, despite evidence that this increase may be slowing or stabilizing,

The views expressed in this article are those of the author and do not necessarily reflect the view of the National Institutes of Health (NIH) or the U.S. Department of Health and Human Services.

Disclosure: None.

Health Behaviors Research Branch, Behavioral Research Program, Division of Cancer Control and Population Sciences, National Cancer Institute, National Institutes of Health, 9609 Medical Center Drive, Room 3E108, Rockville, MD 20892, USA

E-mail address: Susan.Czajkowski@nih.gov

Pediatr Clin N Am 63 (2016) 389–399
http://dx.doi.org/10.1016/j.pcl.2016.02.009
0031-3955/16/$ – see front matter Published by Elsevier Inc.

pediatric.theclinics.com

especially in very young children,[3] obesity in childhood remains a significant behavioral risk factor and an important target of National Institutes of Health (NIH) funding efforts. In addition, wide disparities in obesity rates remain among population subgroups, with minority and low-income children and adolescents showing the highest rates of obesity.[3] Thus, an important focus of pediatric obesity research is identifying and implementing more effective interventions to reduce obesity in vulnerable and underserved groups, such as minority and low-income children and families.

NIH support for childhood obesity research spans the translational spectrum, from basic research on the psychological, behavioral, biological and social processes that characterize early childhood development and present potential targets for obesity-related treatments, to studies that translate knowledge about these processes into obesity-related interventions for children, to efficacy and effectiveness trials, and finally, to dissemination and implementation of treatments in clinical and community settings. NIH research in these areas has undoubtedly contributed, along with efforts at local, state, and national levels, to recent progress in achieving lower obesity levels in young children.[3]

This overview focuses on selected examples of NIH-funded early phase translational studies that use basic behavioral science findings to inform obesity interventions for children at all stages of development, from infancy through adolescence. It is not intended to be comprehensive, because an in-depth review of work in this area is beyond the scope of this article. Instead, by highlighting several promising lines of NIH-supported pediatric obesity research in the basic-to-clinical arena, this article seeks to illustrate how such research can contribute to efforts to reduce childhood obesity and ultimately, the chronic diseases resulting from it.

SUPPORT FROM THE NATIONAL INSTITUTES OF HEALTH FOR BASIC AND EARLY PHASE TRANSLATIONAL BEHAVIORAL RESEARCH IN PEDIATRIC OBESITY

Understanding the basic biological, behavioral, social, and psychological processes that underlie childhood obesity is key to identification of new treatment targets and the development of more effective interventions to tackle this behaviorally based risk factor (see[5] for an excellent overview of basic science findings in pediatric obesity research). Much of the NIH-supported basic behavioral research examining the influence of factors such as cognitive and affective processes, stress and stress reactivity, social relationships and dynamics, and the built environment on obesity-related health behaviors has involved the funding of investigator-initiated grants and Institute-specific research initiatives (see http://www.obesityresearch.nih.gov/ for information and resources related to NIH's obesity research portfolio, strategic plan, and funding opportunities). Recently, however, several large NIH-initiated efforts have been developed that support work in these areas.

National Institutes of Health Basic Behavioral and Social Science Opportunity Network

In recognition of the importance of basic behavioral research to health, the NIH initiated the Basic Behavioral and Social Science Opportunity Network (OppNet) in November 2009 to support research on the underlying basic mechanisms and processes that influence health-related behaviors (available: http://oppnet.nih.gov/).

OppNet has supported several lines of research on the psychological, social, cognitive, and neural mechanisms underlying obesity-related behaviors in children. These endeavors include investigation of the effects of regular exercise on neural circuitry and brain structure, which demonstrated improvements in frontotemporal white matter integrity[6] and alterations in neural circuitry supporting cognitive control[7] in overweight, sedentary children. OppNet-supported research to identify environmental moderators of pediatric weight loss maintenance found that reduced consumption of food eaten away from home was associated with a lower body mass index (BMI) and body fat in children and identified changes in diet quality as a potential mechanism for this effect.[8] Finally, an OppNet-funded project focusing on links between stress, eating behavior, and obesity in low-income children has sought to identify the biologic and behavioral pathways through which stress may affect obesity in children, for example, by potentially increasing sensitivity to food as a reward or reducing ability to delay gratification for food (Lumeng and Miller,[9] principal investigators, 1R01DK098983). Further details on these and other OppNet-funded projects can be found at http://oppnet.nih.gov/ along with relevant funding opportunity announcements related to basic behavioral science research.

Transdisciplinary Research on Energetics and Cancer

The National Cancer Institute's Transdisciplinary Research on Energetics and Cancer (TREC) program aims to reduce cancer linked with obesity, poor diet, and low levels of physical activity by integrating diverse disciplines to find effective interventions across the lifespan (available: https://www.trecscience.org/trec/default.aspx). TREC was established in 2005 in response to a growing body of evidence that obesity plays a role in the development of many types of cancer. In the initial phase of TREC (2005–2010), 4 TREC Research Centers and 1 Coordination Center were funded, each including scientists from multiple disciplines and encompassing projects spanning the basic biology and genetics of behavioral, sociocultural, and environmental influences on nutrition, physical activity, weight, energy balance, energetics, and cancer risk.

Several TREC projects focused on basic and epidemiologic research in children and adolescents that could be used to develop novel obesity-related interventions. For example, a project led by Susan Redline and colleagues at Case Western Reserve University aimed to define the relationship between risk factors, such as insufficient sleep and sleep apnea in children and adolescents, and changes in both weight and biochemical indices of metabolic pathways implicated in cancer to enable development of targeted interventions for high-risk children. Results from this study demonstrated that chronic insufficient sleep duration, measured longitudinally from infancy to middle childhood, is associated with a lower quality diet in children, with children who had the least favorable diets and sleep duration throughout childhood having the highest estimated BMI z-scores, suggesting that sleep duration and diet quality are important intervention targets in efforts to prevent childhood obesity.[10]

In another TREC project, researchers at the University of Southern California TREC Research Center, led by Michael Goran and his team, explored the physiologic, metabolic, genetic, behavioral, and environmental influences on obesity and cancer risk in minority children. One study in this set of projects, which examined the role of neighborhood-level factors on progression toward overweight and obesity in children, found a significant relationship over an 8-year period between traffic density and BMI in a cohort of 3318 children living in multiple communities in Southern California.[11] These findings implicate traffic, a pervasive feature of urban environments, as a major but potentially modifiable risk factor for the development of obesity in children, and thus provide important information to guide the development of future environmentally based pediatric obesity interventions.

Obesity-Related Behavioral Intervention Trials

Research translating basic behavioral science discoveries into new behavioral interventions for behaviorally based risk factors has not been as well-recognized or resourced as similar early phase translational research in the biomedical arena. Especially in the case of obesity, a complex risk factor based on a combination of biological, behavioral, social, psychological, and environmental influences, accelerating early phase translational research is increasingly being viewed as an important area of need.

In response to this need, in 2009 the NIH initiated the Obesity-Related Behavioral Intervention Trials Consortium (ORBIT; available: www.nihorbit.org), a trans-NIH cooperative agreement program led by the National Heart, Lung, and Blood Institute in collaboration with the National Cancer Institute, the National Institute of Diabetes and Digestive and Kidney Diseases, the Eunice Shriver Kennedy National Institute on Child and Human Development, and the NIH Office of Behavioral and Social Sciences Research. The ORBIT consortium consists of interdisciplinary teams of researchers at 7 research sites and a Resource Coordinating Unit, who are developing and testing novel interventions that translate findings from basic research on human behavior (eg, habituation, motivation, habit formation, stress, and social networks) into more effective clinical, community, and population interventions to reduce obesity and alter obesity-related health behaviors (eg, diet, physical activity). Investigators at each site are conducting several types of studies over the 5-year funding period, including formative research, experimental and proof-of-concept studies, and feasibility pilot studies, to identify and test promising new approaches to reducing obesity and improving obesity-related behaviors.

The ORBIT program is notable for the diversity of its targeted populations; many of its studies focus on vulnerable and underserved groups, including Latino and African American adults, African American adolescents, low-income populations, pregnant women, and women beginning the menopausal transition. The interventions being developed to address obesity and obesity-related behaviors in these groups include a wide range of strategies, including promoting small changes in eating behaviors and physical activity, reducing stress-related eating, improving sleep patterns, increasing motivation to adhere to weight loss strategies, and engaging an individual's social networks and communities to encourage physical activity.

Three of the 7 ORBIT sites are focused on children and adolescents: Reynolds and colleagues at Claremont University conducted research to create a novel intervention based on basic behavioral science findings on habit formation and neurocognition to improve nutrition behavior and reduce risk for obesity in adolescents from low-income families. Naar-King and her team at Wayne State conducted an adaptive 6 month intervention with Community Health Workers using a sequential randomized assignment trial (SMART design) that included skills training modules, motivational conversations and contingency management in African American adolescents and their primary caregivers. Finally, Epstein and colleagues at the University of Buffalo conducted a series of studies to translate habituation theory into interventions for pediatric obesity by reducing the variety of less healthy, high energy density foods to lower their intake while simultaneously increasing the variety of healthier, low energy density options to increase their intake. Findings and implications from these studies are discussed in a later section.

The Obesity-Related Behavioral Intervention Trials Model

In addition to the individual ORBIT projects, a major product of the ORBIT consortium has been the development of a framework to guide the behavioral intervention development process. The ORBIT model consists of a phased approach similar to the drug development model, but adapted for behavioral treatment development.[12] It encompasses 2 overarching phases of intervention development, entitled "phase I" (intervention design) and "phase II" (preliminary testing) and each includes 2 distinct subphases. In phase Ia, treatment targets and components are initially defined, including the degree of change in the treatment target needed to demonstrate a clinically meaningful effect in ultimate health outcome. In phase Ib, these components are tested and refined to achieve a well-defined treatment "package." Phase IIa involves "proof-of-concept" testing, which aims to determine if the treatment package can achieve a clinically significant degree of change in the prespecified treatment target; phase IIb involves further pilot testing using larger samples, randomized designs and a determination of feasibility.

Key features of the ORBIT model include (1) an emphasis on beginning with "with the end in mind"; that is, starting with a "significant clinical question" from providers, patients or others intimately involved in the behavioral issues and/or disease processes at hand to ensure that the intervention being developed will ultimately have "real-world" meaning and impact; (2) using basic behavioral science findings to understand the "drivers" of the behavior or disease being addressed, to identify appropriate and modifiable treatment targets, and define essential interventional components; (3) a focus on achieving not just statistically significant, but clinically meaningful, changes in behavioral treatment targets that are tied to prevention or mitigation of disease risk and outcomes; and (4) progression through a series of flexible, increasingly rigorous phases and study designs as the intervention is designed, refined, optimized and tested, culminating in efficacy and effectiveness trials, and ultimately resulting in the dissemination and implementation of an intervention that has a significant impact on clinical endpoints in a clinical and/or community setting.

Science of Behavior Change Common Fund Program

The Science of Behavior Change Program (SOBC; available: https://commonfund.nih. gov/behaviorchange/index) is an NIH Common Fund initiative that promotes basic and early phase translational research on the initiation, personalization, and maintenance of behavior change. Several projects related to pediatric obesity were funded as part of the initial phase of SOBC. An example is work by Lumeng and colleagues[9] that examines relationships among self-regulation, salivary cortisol and alpha amylase, emotional eating behavior, and weight status in low-income toddlers to better understand the biobehavioral mechanisms of excessive childhood weight gain, potentially leading to more effective, novel, targeted prevention approaches (https:// commonfund.nih.gov/behaviorchange/fundedresearch provides information on this and all SOBC funded research projects).

More recently, the SOBC initiated a program of research based on an "experimental medicine approach" to the development of mechanistically based interventions for preventing and treating unhealthy behaviors linked to disease. This approach is congruent with and expands on the ORBIT model's earliest phase (phase I) by providing a detailed set of steps for identifying and validating behaviorally based treatment targets, including (1) identifying a set of putative targets within a psychological or behavioral domain that is implicated in health behavior, (2) leveraging existing or developing new experimental or intervention approaches to engage the targets, (3) identifying or developing appropriate assays (measures) to permit verification of target engagement, and (4) testing the degree to which engaging the targets produces a desired change in health behaviors that lead to clinically significant outcomes or endpoints. One of the projects funded by this program, led by Alison Miller at the

University of Michigan, involves measuring childhood self-regulation targets known to be associated with obesity risk and testing whether intervening on these mechanisms can improve self-regulation and adherence to weight management regimens in school-age low-income children (for more information, see https://commonfund.nih.gov/behaviorchange/fundedresearch).

HIGHLIGHTS OF NATIONAL INSTITUTES OF HEALTH–FUNDED BASIC AND EARLY PHASE TRANSLATIONAL BEHAVIORAL RESEARCH IN CHILDHOOD OBESITY
Infancy and Early Childhood

Infancy through age 5 is acknowledged to be a critical developmental period for forming the preferences and habits that contribute to obesity-related dietary and physical activity behaviors. Basic behavioral research has found, for example, that at an early age, children heavier for their height prefer food to alternative reinforcers[13] and that obese infants find food more reinforcing than their leaner peers.[14]

A better understanding of the underlying biological, behavioral, social, and psychological factors that predict excessive weight gain in very young children is increasingly being seen as an important part of NIH efforts to reduce childhood (and later life) obesity. In November of 2013, the National Institute of Diabetes and Digestive and Kidney Diseases held a Workshop on "The Prevention of Obesity in Infancy and Early Childhood" to identify what is known about preventing obesity in early childhood and what needs to be done to accelerate research targeting this important developmental period. Citing significant gaps in knowledge concerning the basic biological and behavioral factors underlying excessive weight gain in the birth through 2-year age period, Workshop participants recommended that research in this area be accelerated,[9] resulting in release of an National Institute of Diabetes and Digestive and Kidney Diseases–led, trans-NIH program announcement (PAR-14–323) "Understanding Factors in Infancy and Early Childhood (Birth to 24 months) that Influence Obesity Development" (available: http://grants.nih.gov/grants/guide/pa-files/PAR-14-323.html).

The value of basic and early phase translational research in very young children was illustrated in a recent Expert Panel meeting convened by the Office of Behavioral and Social Sciences Research on "Self-regulation of Appetite," held in July 2015 on the NIH campus in Bethesda, Maryland. The meeting included presentations by several researchers who have published extensively on the biological, social, and psychological bases for eating behaviors in infancy and early childhood.

An example of research in this area is that conducted by Mennella and colleagues who have explored the nature and consequences of very early taste preferences, for example, preference for sweet and aversion to bitter tastes, which in an environment rich in added sugars and salt, can lead to overweight and obesity.[15–17]

In a similar vein, Birch and colleagues have examined the importance of early learning in shaping infant and young children's taste preferences, showing that with repeated exposure even initially rejected new foods can become accepted and liked.[18–20] These researchers have also demonstrated the influence of factors such as temperament, self-regulation capacity, and parental feeding on infants' food intake and risk for obesity,[21–23] and have translated this research into a set of responsive parenting practices related to feeding, for example, provision of alternatives to food as "soothing" behaviors for infant fussiness, increased sleep duration, awareness of hunger/fullness cues, use of repeated food exposures, and delay in introducing solid foods. In a pilot study, infants randomized to these responsive parenting interventions were found to have lower weight for length at 1 year,[24] demonstrating the promise of this approach for reducing obesity risk in infants.

Later Childhood and Adolescence

Research elucidating the psychological, social, and cognitive underpinnings of obesity-related behaviors in children and their families, along with research on the design and testing of interventions based on these findings, has resulted in the development of several evidence-based, efficacious treatments for pediatric obesity.[25,26] A particularly fruitful program of research by Epstein and colleagues incorporates both children and their parents in a family-based treatment (FBT) that has been shown to be highly efficacious.[27,28] The approach uses concepts from basic behavioral research, such as contingency contracting, self-monitoring of weight and food intake, mastery of behavior change, behavioral choice theory, and stimulus control management, among others.[29]

Building on the FBT model to address maintenance of weight loss in children, Wilfley and colleagues[30] have developed a social facilitation maintenance treatment that promotes healthy eating and physical activity after the end of active FBT through extended parent and peer support, improvements in body image, and help in responding to teasing, that has been shown to achieve maintenance of some degree of weight loss. Based on further basic behavioral research showing that previous learned behaviors are highly resistant to extinction and continue to exist alongside newly learned behaviors,[31,32] these investigators have enhanced social facilitation maintenance treatment (SFM+) to incorporate the practicing of newly learned behaviors in multiple contexts to ensure long-term establishment of new, healthier eating and activity habits.[33]

Findings from the ORBIT consortium show how translating concepts from basic behavioral research can result in the development of new, innovative approaches to childhood obesity as well as the addition of new components to existing approaches, thereby bolstering their efficacy. For example, Reynolds and colleagues are developing a new intervention based on basic behavioral research on the formation and maintenance of eating habits in low-income adolescents. The investigators used ecological momentary assessment to identify physical, social, and intrapersonal cues associated with consumption of sweetened beverages and sweet and salty snacks among adolescents. Results showed a number of linkages of cues with snack choices; for example, being at school, with friends, and feeling lonely or bored were associated with having unhealthy snacks and drinks, whereas sweetened drink consumption was associated with engaging in physical exercise.[34] These findings provide insights into the eating and activity behaviors of high-risk adolescents that can be incorporated into the development of interventions to disrupt these cue–behavior linkages, which is the goal of this line of research.

An example of using basic behavioral science findings to develop novel approaches that can increase the potency of existing interventions is demonstrated by Epstein and colleagues at the University of Buffalo ORBIT site. This research team used the psychological construct of habituation, based in learning theory, to test the effects of varying foods at the dinner meal to reduce energy intake. Basic research has shown that increasing variety increases energy intake, and repeated consumption of the same food increases habituation to those foods and reduces consumption. In one of the trials conducted by Epstein and colleagues,[35] 24 families with overweight or obese 8- to 12-year-old children and overweight or obese parents were randomly assigned to 6 months of usual FBT or FBT plus reduced variety of high energy-dense foods (FBT + variety). Results showed significant differences between the 2 conditions in child percent overweight and parent BMI, with positive relationships between child zBMI and parent BMI changes and between reductions in food variety of high energy-dense foods and reductions in child zBMI and parent BMI. These pilot data suggest that reducing the variety of high energy dense foods and repeating meals within the context of FBT, both of which are relatively easily implemented within family-based weight loss treatment, may enhance weight loss in children and their parents. Further work is needed to replicate this finding in larger samples and over longer periods of time.

In another ORBIT project, investigators at the Wayne State site conducted an adaptive behavioral treatment for African American adolescents with obesity. In this study, 181 youth ages 12 to 16 years old with primary obesity and their caregiver were first randomized to 3 months of home-based versus office-based delivery of motivational interviewing plus skills building and after 3 months, nonresponders to first phase treatment were rerandomized to continued home-based skills or contingency management. There were no differences in primary outcomes between home-based or office-based delivery or between continued home-based skills or contingency management for nonresponders to first-phase treatment, although families receiving home-based treatment initially attended significantly more sessions in both phases of the trial, and families receiving contingency management attended more sessions in the second phase.[36] Overall, participants demonstrated decreases in percent overweight over the course of the trial (3%), and adolescent executive functioning moderated this effect such that those with higher functioning lost more weight.[36] Results also showed that older children in the home-based contingency monitoring condition showed the greatest decreases in percent overweight, whereas younger adolescents responded more strongly to the home-based skills development sequence.[37] These results suggest it may be important to target psychological factors in obesity treatment, such as executive function, that age is a key variable in tailoring treatments, and that at-home treatment with contingency management may increase session attendance for this vulnerable population.

Research on the relationship of executive functions and eating behavior in childhood and adolescence is a particularly promising avenue of investigation, because a growing body of research has found that the ability to regulate emotions, delay gratification, develop future plans, and avoid or mitigate impulsive actions are critical elements in establishing healthy diets and promoting healthy weight gain from childhood through adolescence and into adulthood. This is exemplified by long-term follow-up studies of Mischel's research on delay of gratification in 4-year-old children in which longer delay of gratification at age 4 has been shown to be related to a lower BMI 30 years later.[38] Several lines of research have investigated the mechanisms through which deficits in executive and neurocognitive function are linked to obesity-related behaviors, such as dietary intake in children and adolescence,[39–41] setting the stage for the development of behavioral interventions designed to improve children's self-regulatory skills.[42]

A related line of research focuses on the relationship of factors, such as food reinforcement, delay discounting and impulsivity to food intake and obesity risk in children.[43–45] Research showing the importance of delay discounting (a measure of impulsivity, ie, the tendency to overvalue present over future rewards) to food intake has led to development of interventions that encourage more forward-looking or prospective thinking in individuals prone to impulsivity as a way to promote better decision-making. One such strategy, episodic future thinking, has been shown to reduce delay discounting and energy intake in adults[46] as well as in overweight/obese children,[47] thus suggesting a new avenue for improving obesity treatment outcomes in children.

SUMMARY/DISCUSSION

Research translating the biological, behavioral, social, and psychological drivers of childhood obesity into novel preventive and therapeutic interventions in children is essential to the development of more effective pediatric obesity interventions. In recognition of this need, the NIH supports investigator-initiated and institute-initiated basic and early phase translational research on pediatric obesity using a variety of funding mechanisms, including investigator-initiated grants and trans-NIH and Institute-initiated research programs.

Funding for basic and translational research has been shown to be critically important in developing successful child and family treatments for obesity, and is necessary for future progress in this area. In addition to overall support for basic-to-clinical translational research, special attention should be paid to designing and testing novel interventions to address the behavioral, social, psychological, and environmental factors that create higher obesity risks and poorer outcomes in minorities and low-income children. Although some of the programs discussed herein have included studies that target these groups, given the continuing high rates of obesity and related diseases in ethnic/racial minorities and low-income children and families, future research should especially focus on developing more effective obesity preventive and therapeutic interventions for these vulnerable subgroups.

Given recent advances in basic behavioral and social sciences research, we are poised for a new era in which new knowledge gained from the basic biological and behavioral sciences can be used to continually "refresh" the pipeline so that more powerful preventive and therapeutic treatments for childhood obesity can be developed, ultimately reducing obesity rates in both children and adults and lowering obesity-related risk for chronic diseases later in life.

REFERENCES

1. Freedman DS, Mei Z, Srinivasan SR, et al. Cardiovascular risk factors and excess adiposity among overweight children and adolescents: the Bogalusa Heart Study. J Pediatr 2007;15:12–7.
2. Taveras EM, Rifas-Shiman SL, Belfort MB, et al. Weight status in the first 6 months of life and obesity at 3 years of age. Pediatrics 2009;123:1177–83.
3. Ogden CL, Carroll MD, Kit BK, et al. Prevalence of childhood and adult obesity in the United States, 2011-2012. JAMA 2014;311:806–14.
4. Boyer BP, Nelson JA, Holub SC. Childhood body mass index trajectories predicting cardiovascular risk in adolescence. J Adolesc Health 2015;56: 599–605.
5. Epstein LH, Wrotniak BH. Future directions for pediatric obesity treatment. Obesity (Silver Spring) 2010;18:S8–12.
6. Schaeffer DJ, Krafft CE, Schwarz NF, et al. An 8-month exercise intervention alters frontotemporal white matter integrity in overweight children. Psychophysiology 2014;51:728–33.
7. Krafft CE, Schwarz NF, Chi L, et al. An eight month randomized controlled exercise trial alters brain activation during cognitive tasks in overweight children. Obesity 2014;22:232–42.
8. Altman M, Holland JC, Lundeen D, et al. Reduction in food away from home Is associated with improved child relative weight and body composition outcomes and this relation Is mediated by changes in diet quality. J Acad Nutr Diet 2015; 115(9):1400–7.
9. Lumeng JC, Taveras EM, Birch L, et al. Prevention of obesity in infancy and early childhood: a National Institutes of Health workshop. JAMA Pediatr 2015;169(5): 484–90.

10. Cespedes EM, Hu FB, Redline S, et al. Chronic insufficient sleep and diet quality: Contributors to childhood obesity. Obesity (Silver Spring) 2016;24(1):184–90.

11. Jerrett M, McConnell R, Chang CC, et al. Automobile traffic around the home and attained body mass index: a longitudinal cohort study of children aged 10-18 years. Prev Med 2010;50(Suppl 1):S50–8.

12. Czajkowski SM, Powell LH, Adler N, et al. From ideas to efficacy: The ORBIT model for developing behavioral treatments for chronic diseases. Health Psychol 2015;34(10):971–82.

13. Kong KL, Feda DM, Elden RD, et al. Origins of food reinforcement in infants. Am J Clin Nutr 2015;101:515–22.

14. Temple JL, Legierski CM, Giacomelli AM, et al. Overweight children find food more reinforcing and consume more energy than do nonoverweight children. Am J Clin Nutr 2008;87(5):1121–7.

15. Drewnowski A, Mennella JA, Johnson SL, et al. Sweetness and food preference. J Nutr 2012;142(6):1142S–8S.

16. Mennella JA, Bobowski NK. The sweetness and bitterness of childhood: Insights from basic research on taste preferences. Physiol Behav 2015;152(Pt B):502–7.

17. Mennella JA, Finkbeiner S, Lipchock SV, et al. Preferences for salty and sweet tastes are elevated and related to each other during childhood. PLoS One 2014;9(3):e92201.

18. Birch LL, Marlin DW. I don't like it; I never tried it: effects of exposure on two-year-old children's food preferences. Appetite 1982;3(4):353–60.

19. Savage JS, Peterson J, Marini M, et al. The addition of a plain or herb-flavored reduced-fat dip is associated with improved preschoolers' intake of vegetables. J Acad Nutr Diet 2013;37(7):954–60.

20. Sullivan SA, Birch LL. Infant dietary experience and acceptance of solid foods. Pediatrics 1994;93(2):271–7.

21. Anzman-Frasca S, Stifter CA, Paul IM, et al. Infant temperament and maternal parenting self-efficacy predict child weight outcomes. Infant Behav Dev 2013; 36(4):494–7.

22. Anzman-Frasca S, Stifter CA, Birch LL. Temperament and childhood obesity risk: a review of the literature. J Dev Behav Pediatr 2012;33:732–45.

23. Birch LL, Fisher JO, Davison KK. Learning to overeat: maternal use of restrictive feeding practices promotes girls' eating in the absence of hunger. Am J Clin Nutr 2003;78:215–20.

24. Paul IM, Savage JS, Anzman SL, et al. Preventing obesity during infancy: a pilot study. Obesity (Silver Spring) 2011;19(2):353–61.

25. Coppock JH, Ridolfi DR, Hayes JF, et al. Current approaches to the management of pediatric overweight and obesity. Curr Treat Options Cardiovasc Med 2014; 16(11):343.

26. Wilfley DE, Tibbs TL, Van Buren DJ, et al. Lifestyle interventions in the treatment of childhood overweight: a meta-analytic review of randomized controlled trials. Health Psychol 2007;26(5):521–32.

27. Epstein LH, Valoski A, Wing RR, et al. Ten-year follow-up of behavioral, family-based treatment for obese children. JAMA 1990;264(19):2519–23.

28. Epstein LH, Paluch RA, Roemmich JN, et al. Family-based obesity treatment: then and now. Twenty-five years of pediatric obesity treatment. Health Psychol 2007;26(4):381–91.

29. Epstein LH, Myers MD, Raynor HA, et al. Treatment of pediatric obesity. Pediatrics 1998;101:554–70.

30. Wilfley DE, Stein RI, Saelens BE, et al. Efficacy of maintenance treatment approaches for childhood overweight: a randomized controlled trial. JAMA 2007; 298(14):1661–73.
31. Bouton ME. Context, ambiguity, and unlearning: Sources of relapse after behavioral extinction. Biol Psychiatry 2002;52(10):976–86.
32. Bouton ME, Westbrook RF, Corcoran KA, et al. Contextual and temporal modulation of extinction: behavioral and biological mechanisms. Biol Psychiatry 2006; 60(4):352–60.
33. Wilfley DE, Van Buren DJ, Theim KR, et al. The use of biosimulation in the design of a novel multilevel weight loss maintenance program for overweight children. Obesity (Silver Spring) 2010;18(S1):S91–8.
34. Grenard JL, Stacy AW, Shiffman S, et al. Sweetened drink and snacking cues in adolescents: a study using ecological momentary assessment. Appetite 2013;67: 61–73.
35. Epstein LH, Kilanowski C, Paluch RA, et al. Reducing variety enhances effectiveness of family-based treatment for pediatric obesity. Eat Behav 2015;17:140–3.
36. Naar-King S, Ellis DA, Idalski Carcone A, et al. Sequential Multiple Assignment Randomized Trial (SMART) to construct weight loss interventions for African American adolescents. J Clin Child Adolesc Psychol 2015;10:1–14.
37. Naar-King S, Ellis D, Jacques-Tiura A, et al. Translating basic behavioral science of learning and motivation into an adaptive community-based obesity treatment for African American Adolescents. Presented at Obesity Week, November 2–7, 2015, Los Angeles, CA.
38. Schlam TR, Wilson NL, Shoda Y, et al. Preschoolers' delay of gratification predicts their body mass 30 years later. J Pediatr 2013;162(1):90–3.
39. Liang J, Matheson BE, Kaye WH, et al. Neurocognitive correlates of obesity and obesity-related behaviors in children and adolescents. Int J Obes (Lond) 2014; 38(4):494–506.
40. Miller AL, Lee HJ, Lumeng JC. Obesity-associated biomarkers and executive function in children. Pediatr Res 2015;77(1–2):143–7.
41. Reinert KRS, Po'e EK, Barkin SL. The relationship between executive function and obesity in children and adolescents: a systematic literature review. J Obes 2013. http://dx.doi.org/10.1155/2013/820956.
42. Miller AL, Horodynski MA, Herb HE, et al. Enhancing self-regulation as a strategy for obesity prevention in Head Start preschoolers: the growing healthy study. BMC Public Health 2012;12:1040.
43. Best JR, Theim KR, Gredysa DM, et al. Behavioral economic predictors of overweight children's weight loss. J Consult Clin Psychol 2012;80:1086–96.
44. Francis LA, Susman EJ. Self-regulation and rapid weight gain in children from age 3 to 12 years. Arch Pediatr Adolesc Med 2009;163:297–302.
45. Seeyave DM, Coleman S, Appugliese D, et al. Ability to delay gratification at age 4 years and risk of overweight at age 11 years. Arch Pediatr Adolesc Med 2009; 163:303–8.
46. Daniel TO, Stanton CM, Epstein LH. The future is now: reducing impulsivity and energy intake using episodic future thinking. Psychol Sci 2013;24(11):2339–42.
47. Daniel TO, Said M, Stanton CM, et al. Episodic future thinking reduces delay discounting and energy intake in children. Eat Behav 2015;18:20–4.

From Bench to Bedside

Understanding Stress-Obesity Research Within the Context of Translation to Improve Pediatric Behavioral Weight Management

Amy F. Sato, PhD*, Amy J. Fahrenkamp, MA

KEYWORDS

- Obesity • Stress • Weight management • Adolescents • Translational research
- Mindfulness

KEY POINTS

- Stress, including chronic stress and acute stress reactivity, is associated with pediatric obesity risk.
- Stress has been associated with weight-related outcomes in basic research, yet translational research is needed to inform the development of pediatric behavioral weight control (BWC) trials.
- Mechanisms through which mindfulness interventions may benefit weight management include reduction of stress, enhancing self-regulatory behaviors, and acceptance of discomfort.
- There is a need for future pediatric BWC research examining mindfulness-based approaches, because these may be useful for decreasing the negative impacts of stress on weight management (eg, eating in response to stress).

A growing body of literature suggests that stress, broadly defined as an individual's negative response to an aversive or threatening stimulus,[1] is one contributor to the development and maintenance of obesity in youth.[2] Stress has been associated with increased food intake and cravings for comfort foods (highly palatable, energy-dense foods) among adults[3] and children.[4,5] The literature on chronic stress and obesity risk, which is based on cross-sectional and longitudinal methodologies, focuses primarily on life stressors. A separate and smaller body of experimental literature has examined the effects of subjective (ie, perceived stress) and objective (eg, cortisol reactivity) acute stress response and obesity risk, including the effects of

The authors have nothing to disclose.
Department of Psychological Sciences, Kent State University, 600 Hilltop Drive, Kent, OH 44242, USA
* Corresponding author.
E-mail address: asato2@kent.edu

Pediatr Clin N Am 63 (2016) 401–423
http://dx.doi.org/10.1016/j.pcl.2016.02.003
0031-3955/16/$ – see front matter © 2016 Elsevier Inc. All rights reserved.

stress reactivity on food intake. To date, however, little has been done to apply this research on stress and obesity risk to inform the development of pediatric BWC interventions.

Standard BWC interventions for pediatric populations generally produce beneficial short-term weight loss outcomes by implementing dietary, physical, and behavioral changes.[6] Compared with the BWC outcomes in school-aged children; however, outcomes for adolescents are less consistently favorable. This is important given that approximately 34% of US adolescents (ages 12–19) are overweight or obese,[7] and that overweight adolescents are at increased risk for a host of negative cardiometabolic[8] and psychosocial[9] consequences. It may be particularly important to consider the impact of stress on weight management during the adolescent period. Adolescence is also a period of increased stress due to a multitude of concurrent psychosocial (eg, changing socioenvironmental contexts and emerging independence) and physiologic (eg, puberty) demands.[10] Furthermore, overweight adolescents endorse higher levels of chronic emotional distress compared with lean adolescents.[11] In addition, income disparities exist in pediatric weight management, in that children and adolescents from low-income households show poorer outcomes in traditional BWC treatment.[12] Low-income populations, who likely experience multiple stressors, may be particularly susceptible to the impact of stress on weight outcomes.[13] To date however, little treatment research has actively addressed stress (eg, stress reactivity and stress-related barriers to treatment engagement) in pediatric weight management.[14]

Translational research is crucial to bridge the body of experimental research in stress and obesity to inform the development and implementation of effective pediatric BWC interventions. The primary aims of this review are, within a translational framework, to

1. Discuss research linking stress (ie, chronic stress and acute stress reactivity) and pediatric obesity
2. Provide examples of ways to integrate the stress-obesity research within pediatric BWC
3. Propose that a mindfulness-based approach may be useful in targeting stress reduction within pediatric BWC

Given that there is a lack of child-specific and adolescent-specific literature in some areas discussed within this review article, findings based on adults samples are integrated to highlight key findings while also serving as a guide for areas in need of further investigation using pediatric samples.

LINKING STRESS AND RISK FOR PEDIATRIC OBESITY: EVIDENCE FROM THE CHRONIC STRESS AND ACUTE STRESS REACTIVITY LITERATURES
Chronic Stress

Chronic stress is linked to increased risk for obesity in adults[14] and youth.[15–18] For example, in a 5-year prospective study of adolescents, persistent perceived stress was associated with higher body mass index (BMI) and waist circumference.[16] Low socioeconomic status (SES),[19] adverse life events (eg, high-crime neighborhood),[20] and parent mental health (eg, maternal depression)[21] are examples of chronic stressors that have been associated with greater weight status.[22]

Consistent with Bronfenbrenner and Vasta's[23] socioecological model of child development, stressors can be understood as spanning from proximal (individual-level and parent-level) to more distal (environmental-level) domains. For example, markers of individual-level stress that have been correlated with higher child weight status have included child psychopathology[24] and weight-related peer victimization.[25] Parent-level chronic stressors, such as maternal depression, parenting stress, and time demands, have also been associated with higher youth weight status.[14,21,26] For example, youth whose parents have many time demands may have fewer meals prepared at home.[26] Parent-child conflict may also exacerbate stress eating or unhealthy behaviors.[27] Environmental-level stressors, such as community violence, may also have an adverse impact on healthy pediatric weight management.[20] SES can be conceptualized as an environmental-level risk that it is associated with poorer health outcomes and greater likelihood of obesity.[19]

Some adolescent populations, such as youth from low-income households and racial/ethnic minority youth, are not only at greater risk for obesity[19] but also more vulnerable to experiencing chronic stress and multiple adverse life events.[10] For example, adolescents from low-SES communities may face greater community-level (eg, neighborhood violence), family-level (eg, financial strain and maternal depression), and individual-level (eg, poor academic achievement and internalizing/externalizing symptoms) stressors, which are known to adversely affect health.[28] Financial strain may also affect food choices by encouraging the purchase of low-cost, energy-dense foods such that adolescents have decreased availability of healthy food choices.[29] Furthermore, low-SES youth may be vulnerable to food insecurity (ie, limited or uncertain availability of nutritionally adequate food due to financial constraints), which has, paradoxically, been associated with increased risk for obesity.[30] Because youth from low-SES backgrounds and racial/ethnic minority youth may be particularly vulnerable to experiencing chronic stress, it may be especially important to integrate an understanding of stress within BWC interventions for these populations.

Acute Stress

Laboratory-based research has examined associations between physiologic and behavioral responses to short-term external stressors and markers of obesity risk. The majority of emerging evidence suggests that laboratory-induced physiologic stress reactivity (eg, cortisol, blood pressure, and heart rate) is positively associated with greater BMI, central fat distribution, and percentage body fat in adults[28] as well as in children and adolescents.[24,31–35] For example, one study showed that changes in perceived stress and heart rate reactivity after a speech task predicted greater BMI percentile and percentage body fat in children, independent of ethnicity, age, and gender.[32] This study was conducted, however, in a predominantly white, middle-class sample of school-aged children (ages 8–12 years); research is needed to examine the generalizability of these findings to overweight/obese youth from low-income households. See **Table 1** for a summary of experimental research that has examined stress reactivity in the context of eating and weight-related outcomes in pediatric samples. Only one of these studies included ethnic/racial minority youth as the majority of their sample, although a majority of adolescent participants were from middle-income households.[33] This study examined the associations between laboratory-induced stress, delayed discounting (impulsivity tendencies), and BMI among urban Chinese adolescents. The results showed that delayed discounting significantly mediated higher levels of stress reactivity and greater BMI.[33] The remaining studies presented in **Table 1** included predominantly white, middle-income to high-income pediatric samples, thus demonstrating the need to examine the relationship between stress and weight management in at-risk minority populations.

A small body of literature shows a positive association between higher levels of visceral (abdominal) fat and higher cardiovascular reactivity.[35] For example, among

Table 1
Experimental research using laboratory-induced stressors to examine stress reactivity in the context of eating and weight-related outcomes among pediatric samples

Reference	Age (y)	Laboratory-induced Stressors	Controls/ Comparison Groups	Stress Reactivity Measures	Objective Outcome Measures	Results
Balantekin & Roemmich,[4] 2012	8–12	3-min speech in front of a video camera, 5-min speech preparation	Within-subjects design in which all participants completed control condition (reading children's magazines for 15-min) and stress condition during separate laboratory visits	• Heart rate • Blood pressure	• BMI z scores for age and gender • Observed coping behaviors: 25-min access to (1) snack foods; (2) television show; and (3) PA equipment (eg, stationary bicycle)	Overall, children watching television more often than any other activity, after social stressor. Children with higher levels of dietary restraint (as measured by DEBQ) and higher stress reactivity had greater food intake than other children completing stressor task.
Barnes et al,[92] 1998	13 and older	• Postural change (3-min) • Video game • Forehead cold stimulation (1-min)	No control condition	• Blood pressure (systolic and diastolic) • Cardiac output	• WTH (upper and lower) • BMI • Triceps skinfold and body surface area	After controlling for BMI and tricep skinfolds, upper WTH had higher stress reactivity (systolic blood pressure) from postural change and video game stressors. Upper WTH also predicted higher stress reactivity (diastolic blood pressure) in postural change in cold stimulation stressors.

Study	Age	Stressor task	Control condition	Stress measure	Outcome measure	Results
Dockray et al,[24] 2009	8–13	TSST-C	No control condition	Salivary cortisol	BMI for age	In girls, higher cortisol reactivity mediated the relationship between depressive symptoms and greater BMI. In boys, there was no significant mediation, but greater depressive symptoms were significantly related to cortisol reactivity and BMI in regression model.
Francis et al,[34] 2013	5–9	TSST-C with speech and mental arithmetic stressor tasks	No control condition	Salivary cortisol	• BMI percentile and z scores for age and gender • Free access to 10 snack foods	In children ages 8–11 y old, higher cortisol reactivity was associated with higher levels of BMI and greater food intake.
Goldbacher et al,[35] 2005	14–16	• Mental arithmetic • Mirror-image tracing • Type A adolescent structured interview • Forehead cooling	No control condition	• Blood pressure (systolic and diastolic) • Heart rate • Cardiac output	• BMI (kg/m^2) • Central adiposity assessed by waist circumference	Overall, higher levels of central adiposity were associated with greater blood pressure and cardiovascular reactivity to stress, even after controlling for overall adiposity.

(continued on next page)

Table 1
(continued)

Reference	Age (y)	Laboratory-induced Stressors	Controls/ Comparison Groups	Stress Reactivity Measures	Objective Outcome Measures	Results
Horsch et al,[57] 2015	7–11	TSST-C	Randomly assigned to 1 of 2 conditions: (1) moderate PA (basketball, running, and climbing stairs); (2) sedentary activity (choice between calm board games, reading books, or drawing). TSST-C followed.	Heart rate	• BMI percentile • Waist circumference • Energy intake from high caloric density snack foods (comfort foods) and low-density foods (healthy food)	Overweight or obese children ate significantly more high-density snack foods than low-density foods, regardless of activity condition. Moderate PA decreased overall food intake among normal weight and overweight/obese children after stressor task.
Lu et al,[33] 2014	12–13	TSST-C	No control condition	Salivary cortisol	• BMI (kg/m^2) • Body fat percentage assessed by InBody 3.0 segmental bio-impedance analyzer • Delayed discounting task	In female adolescents, greater delayed discounting mediated the relationship between higher cortisol reactivity and greater levels of body fat percentage.
Park et al,[41] 2015	14–16	• Mental arithmetic with sequential subtraction • Videotaped speech task into a microphone	No control condition	• Heart rate • Skin conductance level	• BMI z scores for age and gender	Lower heart rate during resting period and after stress were associated with greater BMI among adolescents.

Source	Age	Stress Task	Design	Measures	Results
Roemmich et al,[5] 2003	8–12	5-min videotaped speech with 15-min to prepare	2 d within-subjects design: control condition (reading children's magazines for 20-min) and stress condition (public speaking task)	• Heart rate to determine low-reactive vs high-reactive from median split • Perceived stress: 100-mm VAS (very relaxed to very stressed [worried]) • BMI percentile • Skinfold measurements from subscapular, triceps, suprailiac, abdominal, thigh, and midcalf • Choice behaviors: cycle ergometer or watching television/playing video games	High-reactive children performed shorter durations of PA after speech task. These children also watched more television on the stress day compared with control condition. No interactions were detected with BMI and stress in influencing sedentary or PA behaviors.
Roemmich et al,[93] 2011	8–12	5-min videotaped speech with 5-min to prepare	2 d with stress and control conditions in counterbalanced order; within-subjects design	• Perceived stress assessed by 100-mm VAS from not stressed to very stressed • Body composition (body fat percentage) from skinfolds: subscapular, triceps, abdominal, and midcalf • Free access to 4 snack foods: 2 comfort foods (1 salty, 1 sweet) and 2 healthier foods (1 salty, 1 sweet)	Higher stress reactivity interacting with higher restraint was significantly associated with greater caloric intake, and were more likely to eat comfort foods.
Roemmich et al,[32] 2007	8–12	5-min videotaped speech about the qualities that make a friend; 15-min speech preparation	2 d with stress and control conditions randomized among participants.	• Heart rate • Perceived stress assessed by 100-mm analog scale (very relaxed to very stressed [or worried]) • BMI percentile for age and gender • Skinfolds (subscapular, triceps, suprailiac, abdominal, thigh, and midcalf) • Waist circumference	Greater heart rate reactivity was related to higher levels of BMI percentile and waist circumference, after controlling for baseline heart rate, gender, age, ethnicity, and baseline perceived stress.

(continued on next page)

Table 1
(continued)

Reference	Age (y)	Laboratory-induced Stressors	Controls/ Comparison Groups	Stress Reactivity Measures	Objective Outcome Measures	Results
Roemmich et al,[58] 2002	8–11	5-min videotaped speech with 15-min speech preparation	2 d with stress and control conditions randomized among participants.	• Perceived stress, assessed by 100-mm analog scale (very relaxed to very stress [worried]) • Dietary restraint measured by DEBQ and median split determined high-restraint vs low-restraint	• BMI percentile for age and gender • Body composition from skinfold assessments • Caloric intake of children's 3 highly rated snack foods	High-restraint/high-reactive children ate significant more snack foods in stress condition compared with control condition.
Verdejo-Garcia et al,[94] 2015	12–18	Virtual reality version TSST with speech task	No control condition	• Salivary cortisol • VAS to assess self-reported arousal and stress	Cognitive measures: 2 Cambridge Neuropsychological Test Automated Battery subtests and Iowa gambling task	Higher cortisol reactivity and lower attention abilities resulted from the laboratory stressor reaction in overweight and obese adolescents.

Abbreviations: DEBQ, Dutch Eating Behavior Questionnaire; PA, physical activity; VAS, visual analog scale; WTH, waist-to-hip ratio.

adolescents participating in 4 laboratory stressor tasks – mental arithmetic, interview, mirror-image tracing, and forehead cooling – participants with greater waist circumference showed greater cardiovascular reactivity.[35] These findings are important given that visceral fat is an important predictor for assessing weight gain related to stress.[36] Specifically, an increase in cortisol release is thought to stimulate abdominal weight gain, given that more glucocorticoid receptors reside in humans' abdominal region.[37,38]

Cortisol stress reactivity and adiposity in youth. For example, in 8-year-old to 9-year-old children, greater cortisol reactivity to a standard laboratory stress paradigm (Trier Social Stress Test for Children [TSST-C][36]) was associated with greater BMI percentile.[34] A different research team showed that higher cortisol reactivity to a speech stressor task was positively associated with higher BMI in girls.[24] Although the literature overall suggests a hyper-responsive hypothalamic-pituitary-adrenal (HPA) axis in obese individuals, there are mixed findings within the body of literature on HPA axis dysregulation and cortisol activity in obesity.[39] For example, past research largely suggests that chronic stress in individuals may consequently lead various obesity-related health issues, such as insulin resistance and metabolic syndrome – precursors to type 2 diabetes mellitus.[40] Other research suggests that disrupted HPA axis functioning, as evidence by reduced cardiovascular stress response and altered diurnal pattern and blunted cortisol stress response, are associated with higher adiposity inadolescents.[41] Given emerging evidence that individuals who are overexposed to stressors may show a blunted stress response resulting in decreased cortisol levels and other associated neurobiological dysfunction,[28,42] there is a need to empirically evaluate patterns of cortisol stress reactivity particularly among at-risk youth (eg, low-income or racial/ethnic minority), who are at heightened risk for chronic stress.

UNDERSTANDING CORTISOL EXPOSURE: AN EXPLANATION FOR WHY STRESS IS ASSOCIATED WITH EATING BEHAVIOR AND OBESITY RISK IN ADOLESCENTS

Consistent with a translational research approach that bridges the chasm between stress-obesity experimental research to inform the development of pediatric BWC, researchers must explore possible mechanisms by which heightened stress reactivity and chronic stress may have an impact on weight outcomes. There is a particular need to understand physiologic pathways, particularly given that the majority of available research examining links between exposure to stress and childhood obesity has failed to include such pathways.[28] It is within this context that cortisol exposure, and cortisol reactivity more specifically, is considered.

Cortisol Exposure

Stress may contribute to obesity risk via activation of the HPA axis, specifically the release of glucocorticoids from the adrenal cortex, leading to greater cortisol exposure.[43–45] There are at least 2 pathways through chronic cortisol exposure may affect appetitive regulation and subsequently contribute to greater food intake and obesity risk. First, cortisol may interfere with the sensitization of satiety signals produced by insulin and leptin, thus contributing to decreased efficiency of the leptin system and decreasing the inhibition of food intake.[43] Second, cortisol may contribute to increased secretion of neuropeptide Y, subsequently resulting in increased food intake.[43,44] Excessive cortisol secretion resulting from frequent activation of the HPA axis may, over time, contribute to the development of type 2 diabetes mellitus.[46] In overweight youth, higher serum cortisol is associated with decreased insulin sensitivity[47] and presence of the metabolic syndrome.[48]

Cortisol and Eating

The relationship between stress and eating is bidirectional, with approximately 70% of individuals increasing intake when stressed.[43] Cortisol elevation after stress plays a key role in the model of Reward Based Stress Eating.[43] According to this model, response to stress (eg, threat to self-concept) activates the HPA system and triggers cortisol release. Cortisol acts on the brain reward center and contributes to a negative state of hedonic withdrawal. Intake of highly palatable food can then decrease stress-induced HPA axis activation, presumably through release of endogenous opioids, thereby linking stress-induced eating and weight gain.[43,49] Food choice seems directly affected by stress-induced cortisol release. Specifically, cortisol stress response seems to increase preferences for highly palatable, energy-dense foods (ie, high fat–content and high sugar–content foods) that may provide relief from stress but contribute to positive energy balance and fat storage.[50]

For these reasons, stress-induced eating refers to the notion that (1) increased food intake occurs in response to stress and (2) eating highly palatable foods can shut down stress-induced HPA axis activation and decrease the distress.[43,51] This term is similar to but distinct from emotional eating, which is discussed later and is defined as a behavioral pattern of eating (often overeating) in response to a broad range of negative affect,[52] including tiredness, anger, anxiety, loneliness, tension, boredom, and sadness, without specificity to a particular emotion or mood.[53] Stress-induced eating occurs across the BMI continuum[54]; however, youth and adults who endorse greater eating in response to stress are more likely to be overweight.[55] Given that stress often comes before weight gain in youth and adults,[16,56] a pattern of eating in response to stress may have an important cumulative effect if stress is chronic.

A small but growing number of studies supports the assertion that greater stress-induced cortisol reactivity predicts greater food intake after stress, independent of BMI status.[3,45] For example, women classified as high cortisol reactors consumed more calories after stress than low reactors but ate similar amounts on the nonstress day.[3] There is little research on stress reactivity and food intake in children. Francis and colleagues[34] found that children (not selected for BMI) who showed greater stress-related cortisol release after the TSST-C had higher BMI scores and consumed more calories in the absence of hunger. This research is limited, however, in that food intake was not measured on the nonstress day, hindering the ability to draw conclusions about the effects of the stressor on energy intake. This study also lacked generalizability to other low-income and racial/ethnic minority populations, because the majority of the sample included white children from middle-income families.[34]

Apart from cortisol response, other work recently found that overweight/obese children ate more high-density salty comfort foods after an acute stress task compared with their healthy-weight peers.[57] Finally, Roemmich and colleagues[58] observed that among children not selected for BMI, children with greater perceived stress reactivity and greater dietary restraint ate more snacks after a laboratory stressor. Youth with lower perceived stress consumed the same number of calories on the stress and control days regardless of whether they were high or low on dietary restraint, underscoring the importance of stress reactivity for altering snacking behavior.[58] This finding is interesting given the body of literature suggesting that adults and children who are higher on dietary restraint tend to eat more in response to stress.[3,56,58] Expanding from cognitive abilities required for restrained dieting, lower levels of broader executive functioning skills – including decision making, self-regulation, and inhibitory control – have also been related to greater emotional eating in adults and pediatric samples. In preschoolers with poorer executive functioning and emotion regulation, stress was associated with greater food intake in the absence of hunger.[59] A reciprocal relationship may exist, in that obesity may have an impact on executive functioning abilities. Obese adolescents (ages 14–21) show lower cognitive functioning, higher self-reported disinhibited eating, and lower frontal cortex volume compared with their healthy-weight counterparts.[60] Given that executive function capacities are not fully developed until late adolescence, training overweight/obese adolescents to enhance healthy emotion regulation skills during stress may be crucial to healthy weight management.[59]

IMPLICATIONS OF LABORATORY STRESS-OBESITY RESEARCH FOR THE DEVELOPMENT AND REFINEMENT OF PEDIATRIC BEHAVIORAL WEIGHT CONTROL INTERVENTIONS

Translational research is needed to apply the available laboratory findings regarding the stress-obesity link to inform the development of pediatric BWC interventions. Examples of the these implications include the importance of addressing stress-related barriers to treatment engagement, attending to patterns of emotional eating, and integrating strategies aimed at decreasing physiologic stress reactivity. In addition, it may be especially important to tailor BWC interventions for higher-risk youth (eg, low SES or racial/ethnic minority) to address the chronic stressors that may be acting as barriers to effective weight management.

Addressing Stress-Related Barriers

Stress-related barriers are known to have a negative impact on pediatric weight outcomes[21]; yet few clinical trials clearly focus on reducing relevant stress-related barriers in families. Although many chronic stressors (eg, parental divorce and neighborhood crime) are outside an adolescent's control and it is not possible for clinicians to remove the presence of these stressors, some chronic stressors present logistic barriers to treatment outcomes that can be addressed within clinical trials. For example, time demands and financial constraints (eg, limited income for groceries) present logistic barriers to treatment adherence and overall healthy behaviors. Through the use of community-based intervention sites, one BWC intervention decreased travel burden and made it more feasible for rural families to participate.[61] Other research has incorporated culturally sensitive considerations for African Americans in dietary control treatment and advised tailoring for specific family needs in providing childcare and transportation and in showing empathy for cultural beliefs and familial concerns.[62] These considerations are consistent with a pediatric BWC model that values recognizing and reducing the impact of chronic stress.

Recognizing Patterns of Emotional Eating

One of the implications of the research on stress reactivity and obesity is that within pediatric BWC intervention, it is important to recognize eating patterns that may exacerbate the effects of stress on eating. Emotional eating is hypothesized to be an underlying mechanism linking stress to unhealthy food choices and increased risk for obesity in children.[63] Although findings have been mixed, cross-sectional findings in adults[64] and children[54] suggest that individuals across the BMI continuum who report higher perceived stress engage in greater emotional eating. For example, adults high on emotional eating consumed more sweet high-fat and energy-dense foods after stress regardless of dietary restraint,[65] and they showed a greater cortisol response to an acute stressor than low emotional eaters.[66] One explanation for this is that when stressors activate the neural stress response networks, cognition is biased toward increased emotional activity, executive function is diminished, and behavior occurs in response to formed habits (eg, emotional eating) rather than cognitive appraisal of response options.[50] The effects of glucocorticoid (cortisol) release after stress, which increases motivation to eat, may then simultaneously act in conjunction with the established pattern of emotional eating to further promote food intake.[47] It is important that pediatric BWC interventions address emotional eating. These may include screening for patterns of emotional eating preintervention and designing content to elicit change in emotional eating over the course of intervention, with the goal of decreasing negative reciprocal effects between emotional eating, stress, and weight management outcomes over time. For example, regularly monitoring patterns of emotional eating may help youth recognize and, if appropriate, change this behavior through the use of alternative copies strategies or through deliberate efforts to change the formed habit.

Decreasing Physiologic Stress Reactivity

Related to emotional eating, within BWC intervention it may be helpful to teach regulation of the stress response. Stress, and the subsequent autonomic physiologic response, is an inevitable part of youths' daily lives. Coping behaviors after stress, however, can promote or hinder positive health outcomes. A decrease in an automatic reaction to stress requires improved regulation of stress responses.[67] Relaxation and adaptive coping strategies may be useful for decreasing stress reactivity and quickening recovery from automatic physiologic stress reactivity. For example, obese women were randomly assigned to participate in relaxation training (progressive muscle relaxation and virtual reality relaxation) 4 times per week for 3 weeks. Both intervention groups were compared with 1 control condition, in which women received standard inpatient treatment without relaxation training. Both conditions receiving relaxation training showed significant improvements in decreased emotional eating and increased self-efficacy for controlled eating.[68]

Both subjective (perceived) and objective (physiologic) measures of stress reactivity should be incorporated to assess changes. Typical BWC treatments use weight loss and psychosocial (eg, quality-of-life) outcomes to measure success of the intervention, but other physiologically based outcome measures are not often used in clinical trials. In addition to weight loss, changes in physiologic stress response could be considered a marker of BWC intervention outcome, if stress reduction is an intervention target. For example, baseline and end-of-treatment assessments of salivary cortisol, heart rate, and/or blood pressure response to an acute stressor would allow for an examination of how changes (ideally reductions) in stress reactivity predict weight-related treatment outcomes or changes in other behaviors, such as emotional eating. Helping overweight/obese youth develop coping strategies to adaptively respond to stressors may increase their capabilities to self-regulate their physiologic stress responses. One possibility for teaching coping skills and, potentially, decreasing physiologic stress response within the context of BWC intervention may be through the integration of mindfulness-based approaches.

MINDFULNESS: AN APPROACH FOR REDUCING STRESS AND IMPROVING OUTCOMES WITHIN THE CONTEXT OF PEDIATRIC BEHAVIORAL WEIGHT CONTROL

Broadly, characteristics of mindfulness interventions include nonjudgment, acceptance-based coping strategies, behavioral awareness, and attention to daily living.[69] Although findings have been mixed (see Olson and Emery for review[69]), mindfulness-based interventions have demonstrated promising results in adult eating and weight-control interventions.[70–76] For example, mindfulness-based interventions have been shown to reduce binge eating,[70,73,74] emotional eating,[70] disinhibited eating,[75,76] and stress reactivity in adults.[71] These interventions have varying levels of integration of approaches from empirically supported mindfulness-based interventions, such as dialectical behavior therapy,[77] acceptance and commitment therapy,[78] and mindfulness-based stress reduction (MBSR).[67] Mindfulness-based interventions have also been explored for some pediatric health conditions,[79,80] yet no known mindfulness-based interventions have been incorporated into pediatric BWC clinical trials. Previous treatment research primarily focused on psychosocial outcomes from pediatric mindfulness-based interventions.[81,82] For example, school-based interventions with school-aged children and adolescents show benefits of decreased stress and psychological symptoms from mindfulness-based strategies.[81] Mindfulness-based interventions for low-income and minority youth similarly demonstrated outcomes of decreased stress and psychiatric symptoms.[83] Clinical research is still needed, however, to better understand how mindfulness-based strategies may benefit pediatric weight management. Although a thorough discussion of all potential mechanisms is past the scope of this review, 3 potential mechanisms through which mindfulness may benefit weight management, including reduction of stress, enhancing self-regulatory behaviors, and acceptance of discomfort, are considered. Findings from a recent systematic review suggest that there is a need for greater clarity regarding whether change specifically in level of mindfulness is a mechanism responsible for weight loss and point to a need for further research to explore psychological, biological, and behavioral mechanisms through which mindfulness is associated with weight loss.[69]

Reduction of Stress and Eating in Response to Stress

First, mindfulness-based interventions may have a beneficial effect on weight management through reduction of stress, in particular stress reactivity and eating in response to stress. Higher stress reactivity, greater dietary restraint, and nonawareness of physiologic states may lead to overeating and stress eating.[84] Learning to respond to external stressors with greater awareness and emotional regulation skills is anticipated to lessen habitual reactions to stress and stress eating.[85] Literature on MBSR, a validated group-based intervention,[67] suggests that this approach may have beneficial effects in terms of stress reduction. Mindfulness in MBSR is defined as "moment-to-moment nonjudgmental awareness." Through regular meditative practice and nonjudgmental awareness of the present moment, MBSR participants are taught to more effectively respond to stress with adaptive coping strategies.[39,67]

A growing body of adult literature (**Table 2**) suggests that components of MBSR may have a beneficial effect within the context of weight management.[69] For example, MBSR combined with a stress-eating intervention led to reductions in perceived stress, stress eating, and short-term weight loss among overweight adults.[86] Similarly, overweight/obese women who received an intervention combining components from MBSR, mindfulness-based cognitive therapy (MBCT), and mindfulness-based eating awareness training (MB-EAT) showed significant reductions in cortisol awakening response (CAR) and maintained weight compared with the control group, who gained weight and showed no significant CAR reduction.[71] Together, these findings suggest that mindfulness-based interventions may have the capacity to decrease subjective and objective markers of stress and may have beneficial effects on weight management.

Table 2
Mindfulness interventions incorporating mindfulness-based stress reduction components to improve adult weight management

Reference	Sample Characteristics	Intervention	Assessment Time Points	Main Outcomes
Dalen et al,[70] 2010	• n =10 Obese adults (7 women) • BMI = 30 or above (mean = 36.9, SD = 6.2)	MEAL intervention • 6-wk, 2-h sessions each week • Daily meditation, meditation paired with eating (eg, noticing hunger satiety cues, food cravings, emotional states) • Group sessions included walking, eating, and sitting meditations, yoga, and discussions. • No control condition	Baseline, 12-wk postintervention, and 3-mo follow-up	MEAL intervention produced significant weight loss in all participants on completion of intervention. Significant increases in mindfulness, cognitive restraint were also shown on completion of intervention and at 3-mo follow-up assessment. Participants showed decreased disinhibited eating, uncontrolled eating, binge eating, and perceived stress at intervention completion and follow-up.
Daubenmier et al,[71] 2011	• n = 47 Overweight/obese women • Mean BMI = 31.2 • 62% White, 15% Hispanic/Latino, 15% Asian/Pacific Islander, and 9% other	Mindfulness intervention incorporating MBSR, MBCT, and MB-EAT: • 4-mo, 9 weekly sessions, 2.5-h each • 7-h silent day • Sessions included body scans, guided meditation (eg, walking, sitting, eating), 3-min breathing space (MBCT), and discussions • 30-min at-home practice of formal and informal meditation • Treatment condition compared with wait-list control: participants randomized to condition	Baseline, postintervention	Participants in treatment intervention showed significant improvements in mindfulness and decreases in anxiety levels and eating from external cues in environment. Intervention and wait-list control did not significantly differ in weight change or CAR; however, obese participants in intervention showed significant CAR reductions and maintained weight from baseline to post-treatment assessment.

Study	Sample	Intervention	Assessment	Results
Kearney et al,[72] 2012	• n = 48 Veterans, excluding for major psychiatric diagnoses • Mean BMI = 29.4 (range from 28.0 to 30.8)	MBSR • 8-wk intervention, 2 ½-h weekly sessions • One silent day • Sessions included formal and informal meditation practices (eg, body scans, walking and sitting meditation, yoga). • Participants encouraged formal meditation practices outside sessions, 45-min each day for 6 d each wk as well as mindfulness daily living (eg, eating, driving). • No control condition	Baseline, postintervention, 4-mo follow-up	No significant changes were detected in self-reported uncontrolled eating, emotional eating, or food intake from baseline to postintervention assessments. Correlations, however, showed greater mindfulness associated with decreased emotional eating and uncontrolled eating. MBSR participation also produced significant decreases in depressive symptoms and increases in mindfulness.
Kristeller & Hallett,[73] 1999	• n = 18 Obese women • Mean age = 46.5 (SD =10.5), ranging from 25 to 62 • Mean BMI = 40.33 (ranging from 28 to 52)	6-wk intervention for BED • 7 Sessions over 6-wk • Sessions targeted mindfulness training involving formal daily meditations, eating meditations, informal daily meditations, and discussions and review of treatment progress.	Baseline (3-wk preintervention), 3-wk follow-up	Women reported a decreased frequency and intensity of binges and depressive and anxiety symptoms. Decreased frequency of binges remained at 3-wk follow-up assessment. Significant improvements in mindfulness, perceptions of eating control, and hunger and satiety cues at postintervention assessment. BMI change was not reported in this pilot study.
Kristeller et al,[74] 2014	• n =140 Overweight/obese adults (12% men) • Mean age = 46.6 (ranging from 20 to 74) • Mean BMI = 40.26 (ranging from 26 to 78)	MB-EAT for binge-eating • 12 Group sessions (9 weekly sessions, 3 monthly booster sessions) • Sessions (1 ½-h) involved guided meditation practices focused on eating awareness and emotional states triggering eating behaviors. • Broader meditation practices included body awareness, yoga, and self-acceptance. • Participants randomly assigned to 1 of 3 conditions: (1) MB-EAT; (2) psychoeducational and cognitive-behavioral; and (3) wait-list control condition	Baseline, 1-mo postintervention, and follow-up assessment occurring between 4 and 6 mo postintervention	Although no significant group differences were found, MB-EAT and psychoeducation/cognitive-behavioral intervention groups produced significant decreases in reported binge eating. MB-EAT group showed larger magnitude of effects regarding reactivity to food and disinhibited eating. Weight loss was not the focus of this intervention, and no significant differences in weight change were found between intervention groups.

(continued on next page)

Table 2
(*continued*)

Reference	Sample Characteristics	Intervention	Assessment Time Points	Main Outcomes

Miller et al,[75] 2014,[75] 2012[76]	• n = 52 Adults with type 2 diabetes mellitus with no required insulin therapy
	• Ages 35–65
		2 Interventions
		• Both 3-mo manualized interventions
		• 8 Weekly and 2 biweekly group sessions
		• Participants randomly assigned to 1 of 2 intervention groups.
		1. MB-EAT for diabetes
		  • Weekly sessions involving guided meditations regarding eating
		  • Awareness training for hunger cues, stress, and food choices
		2. SC diabetes self-management education
		  • Derived from social cognitive theory and meaningful learning
		  • Goals to increase knowledge of diabetes, self-efficacy, and self-management
			Baseline, postintervention, -month and 3-mo follow-up assessments	Both intervention groups showed significant diabetes self-management (glycemia), weight loss, decreased depressive symptoms, increased self-efficacy in eating, and decreased disinhibited eating. MB-EAT for diabetes showed significantly higher changes in increased mindfulness compared with SC group; however, SC group showed a significantly higher increase in fruit/vegetable consumption.

Smith et al,[95] 2006	• n = 25 (80% Women) • Mean age = 47.8, SD = 13.1 • Mean BMI = 27.9, SD = 7.4	Modified eating-focused MBSR intervention • 8-wk MBSR intervention with 1 full-day silent retreat • Weekly sessions lasted 3-h • Breathing, body scans, formal and informal meditations, yoga, and discussions • Focus on mindful eating exercises, awareness, and mindful choices of healthy foods • No control condition	Baseline, postintervention	Overall, participants in intervention showed significant reductions in reported binge eating, anxiety, and depressive symptoms as well as significant increases in mindfulness and self-acceptance from baseline to postintervention.

Abbreviations: BED, binge-eating disorder; MEAL, Mindful Eating and Living; SC, Smart Choices.

Improved Self-regulatory Behaviors

Self-regulatory health behaviors (eg, dietary self-monitoring, decreasing caloric intake, and increasing physical activity) are standard components of BWC interventions, and these behaviors predict favorable treatment outcome. For example, low-income adolescents who consistently self-monitored lost more weight and had better attendance compared with those who did not consistently monitor their progress.[87] Mindfulness may enhance regulatory behaviors needed for successful weight loss.[69] For example, mindfulness intervention in the form of eating meditations helped individuals gain awareness of hunger and satiety cues and food sensitivity.[74] Mindfulness interventions may be particularly helpful for individuals experiencing stress and fatigue, because these experiences may deplete cognitive resources and make self-regulation of weight-related behaviors, such as eating, more difficult in times of distress. It is also plausible that implementing eating awareness interventions while also reducing caloric intake may diminish the paradoxic pattern of dietary restraint. Dietary restraint is often part of weight loss but also leads to overeating when stressed.[88] Recent work implemented MB-EAT, an intervention derived from MBSR and literature on self-regulatory eating behavior, among a sample of adults with binge-eating disorder.[74] Results showed greater mindfulness practice associated with lower self-reported disinhibition, lower levels of binge eating, and weight loss.[74] Eating-related meditation and broader eating awareness might be incorporated into efforts to reduce caloric intake, for example, by choosing smaller portion sizes to gauge hunger cues throughout a meal.[74]

Increased Acceptance of Discomfort

Mindfulness may also serve to facilitate weight management by enhancing tolerance of the discomfort that is often experienced during the process of weight loss. It is common that individuals participating in BWC intervention experience some level of discomfort due to hunger (eg, discomfort associated with food cravings) and physical activity (eg, discomfort associated with muscle soreness). Outside of physical discomfort, individuals may experience psychological discomfort (eg, feeling self-conscious when making different food choices when eating with friends). Mindfulness-based interventions promote acceptance of uncomfortable feelings, or undesirable situations, as opposed to avoidant coping strategies.[67] In this way, mindfulness training may provide individuals with greater tolerance for discomfort (a source of stress) when framed within their weight loss goals.

Nonjudgmental acceptance and awareness may also help individuals when drawbacks occur in their weight loss goals. Consuming non-nutritional foods, eating more than daily caloric intake goals, or missing planned physical activity are setbacks that regularly occur when trying to lose weight. When individuals consume non-nutritional foods, instead of feeling guilty, a mindfulness stance promotes nonjudgment and acceptance of difficulties throughout the treatment.[67,69,89] Nonjudgmental awareness in weight control setbacks may be beneficial in allowing continued progress toward weight management goals.

FUTURE DIRECTIONS: ADDRESSING THE ROLE OF STRESS TO INFORM THE DEVELOPMENT OF PEDIATRIC BEHAVIORAL WEIGHT CONTROL INTERVENTION

Given the body of basic science research suggesting that stress is important for eating and weight management outcomes, future research is needed to (1) measure the impact of stress on response to intervention and (2) develop and refine pediatric BWC interventions that clearly target a reduction in stress. For example, it would be useful for future BWC interventions to include both subjective (perceived stress) and objective (eg, cortisol and heart rate) indicators of stress within the context of pediatric BWC interventions. This kind of measurement strategy would be helpful in addressing questions, such as whether baseline level of chronic stress (child level or family level) has an impact on response to intervention; whether markers of physiologic stress (eg, diurnal cortisol) or perceived stress (eg, as rated by self-report of global stress) more strongly predict intervention adherence and/or outcome; or whether stress response (including stress reactivity and coping in response to stress) changes over the course of intervention.

Additional investigation is also needed to examine the potential utility of integrating mindfulness-based approaches as a method of targeting stress reduction within BWC control intervention for overweight/obese adolescents. Growing child/adolescent literature supports mindfulness interventions for a range of outcomes (eg, anxiety and depression) in youth.[90] Emerging research supports the use of mindfulness interventions with low-income and minority youth, including those with chronic health conditions (eg, pediatric HIV)[83] and suggests potential for improved physiologic outcomes, such as blood pressure reduction in adolescent minority youth.[90] Although stress is thought to be salient during this developmental window, the integration of mindfulness-based approaches may be especially relevant to adolescents (eg, low-SES youth and racial/ethnic minorities) at highest risk of chronic stress.

One option for integrating mindfulness strategies within the context of standard BWC content may be through the implementation of MBSR skills. Interventions, including MBSR skills, have been shown to yield stress reduction as well as other beneficial health outcomes among pediatric samples.[82] For example, MBSR programs led to positive outcomes among youth with chronic pain[79] and psychiatric symptoms.[82] This intervention model has also been successfully implemented with adolescents. For example, MBSR for teens led to improved mindfulness, improved affect regulation, and decreased reactivity to external stressors.[85] Positive effects of MBSR for teens were also seen among low-income Hispanic adolescents.[91] Future research is needed to explore whether MBSR may be suitable for augmenting BWC among overweight/obese adolescents.

REFERENCES

1. De Vriendt T, Moreno LA, De Henauw S. Chronic stress and obesity in adolescents: scientific evidence and methodological issues for epidemiological research. Nutr Metab Cardiovasc Dis 2009;19(7):511–9.
2. Wilson SM, Sato AF. Stress and paediatric obesity: what we know and where to go. Stress Health 2014;30(2):91–102.
3. Epel E, Lapidus R, McEwen B, et al. Stress may add bite to appetite in women: a laboratory study of stress-induced cortisol and eating behavior. Psychoneuroendocrinology 2001;26(1):37–49.
4. Balantekin KN, Roemmich JN. Children's coping after psychological stress. Choices among food, physical activity, and television. Appetite 2012;59(2):298–304.
5. Roemmich JN, Gurgol CM, Epstein LH. Influence of an interpersonal laboratory stressor on youths' choice to be physically active. Obes Res 2003;11(9):1080–7.
6. Luttikhuis O, Baur L, Jansen H, et al. Interventions for treating obesity in children. Cochrane Database Syst Rev 2009;(1):CD001872.
7. Ogden CL, Carroll MD, Kit BK, et al. Prevalence of obesity and trends in body mass index among US children and adolescents, 1999-2010. JAMA 2012; 307(5):483–90.

8. Weiss R, Dziura J, Burgert TS, et al. Obesity and the metabolic syndrome in children and adolescents. N Engl J Med 2004;350(23):2362–74.
9. Zeller MH, Roehrig HR, Modi AC, et al. Health-related quality of life and depressive symptoms in adolescents with extreme obesity presenting for bariatric surgery. Pediatrics 2006;117(4):1155–61.
10. Goodman E, McEwen BS, Dolan LM, et al. Social disadvantage and adolescent stress. J Adolesc Health 2005;37(6):484–92.
11. Mellin AE, Neumark-Sztainer D, Story M, et al. Unhealthy behaviors and psychosocial difficulties among overweight adolescents: the potential impact of familial factors. J Adolesc Health 2002;31(2):145–53.
12. Baxter KA, Ware RS, Batch JA, et al. Predicting success: factors associated with weight change in obese youth undertaking a weight management program. Obes Res Clin Pract 2011;7:e147–54.
13. Burke NJ, Hellman JL, Scott BG, et al. The impact of adverse childhood experiences on an urban pediatric population. Child Abuse Negl 2011;35(6):408–13.
14. Koch FS, Sepa A, Ludvigsson J. Psychological stress and obesity. J Pediatr 2008;153(6):839–44.
15. Block JP, He Y, Zaslavsky AM, et al. Psychosocial stress and change in weight among US adults. Am J Epidemiol 2009;170(2):181–92.
16. van Jaarsveld CH, Fidler JA, Steptoe A, et al. Perceived stress and weight gain in adolescence: a longitudinal analysis. Obesity (Silver Spring) 2009;17(12):2155–61.
17. Mellbin T, Vuille JC. Rapidly developing overweight in school children as an indicator of psychosocial stress. Acta Paediatr Scand 1989;78(4):568–75.
18. Yin Z, Davis CL, Moore JB, et al. Physical activity buffers the effects of chronic stress on adiposity in youth. Ann Behav Med 2005;29(1):29–36.
19. Kendzor DE, Caughy MO, Owen MT. Family income trajectory during childhood is associated with adiposity in adolescence: a latent class growth analysis. BMC Public Health 2012;12:611–9.
20. Lumeng JC, Appugliese D, Cabral HJ, et al. Neighborhood safety and overweight status in children. Arch Pediatr Adolesc Med 2006;160:25–31.
21. Garasky S, Stewart S, Gundersen C, et al. Family stressors and child obesity. Soc Sci Res 2009;38:755–66.
22. Daddis C. Desire for increased autonomy and adolescents' perceptions of peer autonomy: "everyone else can; why can't I? Child Dev 2011;82(4):1310–26.
23. Bronfenbrenner U, Vasta R, editors. Six theories of child development: revised formulations and current issues. London: Jessica Kingsley Publishers; 1992. p. 187–249.
24. Dockray S, Susman EJ, Dorn LD. Depression, cortisol reactivity, and obesity in childhood and adolescence. J Adolesc Health 2009;45(4):344–50.
25. Hayden-Wade HA, Stein RI, Ghaderi A, et al. Prevalence, characteristics, and correlates of teasing experiences among overweight children vs. non- overweight peers. Obes Res 2005;13(8):1381–92.
26. Hearst MO, Sevcik S, Fulkerson JA, et al. Stressed out and overcommitted! The relationships between time demands and family rules and parents' and their child's weight status. Health Educ Behav 2012;39(4):446–54.
27. Skouteris H, McCabe M, Ricciardelli LA, et al. Parent–child interactions and obesity prevention: a systematic review of the literature. Early Child Dev Care 2012;182(2):153–74.
28. Gundersen C, Mahatmya D, Garasky S, et al. Linking psychosocial stressors and childhood obesity. Obes Rev 2011;12(5):e54–63.

29. Ver Ploeg M, Breneman V, Farriang T, et al. Access to affordable and nutritious food – measuring and understanding food deserts and their consequences: report to congress. Administrative Publication; 2009. p. 1–160. AP-036.

30. Crawford PB, Webb KL. Unraveling the paradox of concurrent food insecurity and obesity. Am J Prev Med 2011;40(2):274–5.

31. Epel ES, McEwen B, Seeman T, et al. Stress and body shape: stress-induced cortisol secretion is consistently greater among women with central fat. Psychosom Med 2000;62(5):623–32.

32. Roemmich JN, Smith JR, Epstein LH, et al. Stress reactivity and adiposity of youth. Obesity (Silver Spring) 2007;15(9):2303–10.

33. Lu Q, Tao F, Hou F, et al. Cortisol reactivity, delay discounting and percent body fat in Chinese urban young adolescents. Appetite 2014;72:13–20.

34. Francis LA, Granger DA, Susman EJ. Adrenocortical regulation, eating in the absence of hunger and BMI in young children. Appetite 2013;64:32–8.

35. Goldbacher EM, Matthews KA, Salomon K. Central adiposity is associated with cardiovascular reactivity to stress in adolescents. Health Psychol 2005;24(4):375–84.

36. Brambilla P, Bedogni G, Heo M, et al. Waist circumference-to-height ratio predicts adiposity better than body mass index in children and adolescents. Int J Obes (Lond) 2013;37(7):943–6.

37. Drapeau V, Therrien F, Richard D, et al. Is visceral obesity a physiological adaptation to stress? Panminerva Med 2001;43:1–7.

38. Kirschbaum C, Karl-Martin P, Hellhammer DH. The 'trier social stress test' - a tool for investigating psychobiological stress responses in a laboratory setting. Neuropsychobiology 1993;28:76–81.

39. Incollingo Rodriguez AC, Epel ES, White ML, et al. Hypothalamic-pituitary-adrenal axis dysregulation and cortisol activity in obesity: a systematic review. Psychoneuroendocrinology 2015;62:301–18.

40. Pervanidou P, Chrousos GP. Metabolic consequences of stress during childhood and adolescence. Metabolism 2012;61(5):611–9.

41. Park AE, Huynh P, Schell AM, et al. Relationship between obesity, negative affect and basal heart rate in predicting heart rate reactivity to psychological stress among adolescents. Int J Psychophysiol 2015;97(2):139–44.

42. Gunnar M, Quevedo K. The neurobiology of stress and development. Annu Rev Psychol 2007;58:145–73.

43. Adam TC, Epel ES. Stress, eating and the reward system. Physiol Behav 2007;91(4):449–58.

44. Bjorntorp P. Do stress reactions cause abdominal obesity and comorbidities? Obes Rev 2001;2(2):73–86.

45. Newman E, O'Connor DB, Conner M. Daily hassles and eating behaviour: the role of cortisol reactivity status. Psychoneuroendocrinology 2007;32(2):125–32.

46. Rosmond R. Stress induced disturbances of the HPA axis: a pathway to Type 2 diabetes? Med Sci Monit 2003;9(2):RA35–9.

47. Adam TC, Hasson RE, Ventura EE, et al. Cortisol is negatively associated with insulin sensitivity in overweight latino youth. J Clin Endocrinol Metab 2010;95(10):4729–35.

48. Weigensberg MJ, Toledo-Corral CM, Goran MI. Association between the metabolic syndrome and serum cortisol in overweight Latino youth. J Clin Endocrinol Metab 2008;93(4):1372–8.

49. Dallman MF, Pecoraro N, Akana SF, et al. Chronic stress and obesity: a new view of "comfort food. Proc Natl Acad Sci U S A 2003;100(20):11696–701.

50. Dallman MF. Stress-induced obesity and the emotional nervous system. Trends Endocrinol Metab 2010;21(3):159–65.
51. Bjorntorp P, Rosmond R. Obesity and cortisol. Nutrition 2000;16(10):924–36.
52. Thayer RE. Calm energy: how people regulate mood with food and exercise: how people regulate mood with food and exercise. Oxford (MS): Oxford University Press; 2001.
53. Faith MS, Allison DB, Geliebter A. Emotional eating and obesity: theoretical considerations and practical recommendations. In: Dalton S, editor. Overweight and weight management: the health professional's guide to understanding and treatment. Gaithersburg (MD): Aspen; 1995. p. 439–65.
54. Nguyen-Rodriguez ST, Chou CP, Unger JB, et al. BMI as a moderator of perceived stress and emotional eating in adolescents. Eat Behav 2008;9(2): 238–46.
55. Ozier AD, Kendrick OW, Leeper JD, et al. Overweight and obesity are associated with emotion- and stress-related eating as measured by the eating and appraisal due to emotions and stress questionnaire. J Am Diet Assoc 2008;108(1):49–56.
56. Greeno CG, Wing RR. Stress-induced eating. Psychol Bull 1994;115(3):444–64.
57. Horsch A, Wobmann M, Kriemler S, et al. Impact of physical activity on energy balance, food intake and choice in normal weight and obese children in the setting of acute social stress: a randomized controlled trial. BMC Pediatr 2015; 15:12.
58. Roemmich JN, Wright SM, Epstein LH. Dietary restraint and stress-induced snacking in youth. Obes Res 2002;10(11):1120–6.
59. Pieper JR, Laugero KD. Preschool children with lower executive function may be more vulnerable to emotional-based eating in the absence of hunger. Appetite 2013;62:103–9.
60. Maayan L, Hoogendoorn C, Sweat V, et al. Disinhibited eating in obese adolescents is associated with orbitofrontal volume reductions and executive dysfunction. Behav Psychol 2011;19:1382–7.
61. Janicke DM, Sallinen BJ, Perri MG, et al. Comparison of parent-only vs family-based interventions for overweight children in underserved rural settings: outcomes from project STORY. Arch Pediatr Adolesc Med 2008;162(12):1119–25.
62. Di Noia J, Furst G, Park K, et al. Designing culturally sensitive dietary interventions for African Americans: review and recommendations. Nutr Rev 2013; 71(4):224–38.
63. Michels N, Sioen I, Braet C, et al. Stress, emotional eating behaviour and dietary patterns in children. Appetite 2012;59(3):762–9.
64. Tomiyama AJ, Dallman MF, Epel ES. Comfort food is comforting to those most stressed: evidence of the chronic stress response network in high stress women. Psychoneuroendocrinology 2011;36(10):1513–9.
65. Oliver G, Wardle J, Gibson EL. Stress and food choice: a laboratory study. Psychosom Med 2000;62(6):853–65.
66. Raspopow K, Abizaid A, Matheson K, et al. Psychosocial stressor effects on cortisol and ghrelin in emotional and non-emotional eaters: influence of anger and shame. Horm Behav 2010;58(4):677–84.
67. Kabat-Zinn J. Full catastrophe living: using the wisdom of your body and mind to face stress, pain, and illness. New York: Bantam Books; 1990.
68. Manzoni GM, Pagnini F, Gorini A, et al. Can relaxation training reduce emotional eating in women with obesity? An exploratory study with 3 months of follow-up. J Am Diet Assoc 2009;109(8):1427–32.

69. Olson KL, Emery CF. Mindfulness and weight loss: a systematic review. Psychosom Med 2015;77(1):59–67.
70. Dalen J, Smith BW, Shelley BM, et al. Pilot study: mindful eating and living (MEAL): weight, eating behavior, and psychological outcomes associated with a mindfulness-based intervention for people with obesity. Complement Ther Med 2010;18(6):260–4.
71. Daubenmier J, Kristeller J, Hecht FM, et al. Mindfulness intervention for stress eating to reduce cortisol and abdominal fat among overweight and obese women: an exploratory randomized controlled study. J Obes 2011;2011:651936.
72. Kearney DJ, Milton ML, Malte CA, et al. Participation in mindfulness-based stress reduction is not associated with reductions in emotional eating or uncontrolled eating. Nutr Res 2012;32(6):413–20.
73. Kristeller JL, Hallett CB. An exploratory study of a meditation-based intervention for binge eating disorder. J Health Psychol 1999;4(3):357–63.
74. Kristeller J, Wolever RQ, Sheets V. Mindfulness-based eating awareness training (MB- EAT) for binge eating: a randomized clinical trial. Mindfulness 2014;5(3):282–97.
75. Miller CK, Kristeller JL, Headings A, et al. Comparison of a mindful eating intervention to a diabetes self-management intervention among adults with type 2 diabetes: a randomized controlled trial. Health Educ Behav 2014;41(2):145–54.
76. Miller CK, Kristeller JL, Headings A, et al. Comparative effectiveness of a mindful eating intervention to a diabetes self-management intervention among adults with type 2 diabetes: a pilot study. J Acad Nutr Diet 2012;112(11):1835–42.
77. Linehan M, Dexter-Mazza E. Dialectical behavior therapy for borderline personaity disorder. In: Barlow D, editor. Clinical handbook of psychological disorders. 4th edition. New York: Guilford Press; 2008. p. 394–461.
78. Hayes SC, Strosahl KD, Wilson KG. Acceptance and commitment therapy: an experiential approach to behavior change. New York: Guilford Press; 1999.
79. Thompson M, Gauntlett-Gilbert J. Mindfulness with children and adolescents: effective clinical application. Clin Child Psychol Psychiatry 2008;13(3):395–407.
80. Zoogman S, Goldberg SB, Hoyt WT, et al. Mindfulness interventions with youth: a meta-analysis. Mindfulness 2014;6(2):290–302.
81. Greenberg MT, Harris AR. Nurturing mindfulness in children and youth: current state of research. Child Development Perspectives 2011;6(2):161–6.
82. Biegel GM, Brown KW, Shapiro SL, et al. Mindfulness-based stress reduction for the treatment of adolescent psychiatric outpatients: a randomized clinical trial. J Consult Clin Psychol 2009;77(5):855–66.
83. Sibinga EM, Kerrigan D, Stewart M, et al. Mindfulness- based stress reduction for urban youth. J Altern Complement Med 2011;17(3):213–8.
84. Alberts HJ, Thewissen R, Raes L. Dealing with problematic eating behaviour. The effects of a mindfulness-based intervention on eating behaviour, food cravings, dichotomous thinking and body image concern. Appetite 2012;58(3):847–51.
85. Baer RA. Mindfulness-based treatment approaches: clinician's guide to evidence base and applications. Waltham (MA): Elsevier; 2014.
86. Corsica J, Hood MM, Katterman S, et al. Development of a novel mindfulness and cognitive behavioral intervention for stress-eating: a comparative pilot study. Eat Behav 2014;15(4):694–9.
87. Kirschenbaum DS, Germann JN, Rich BH. Treatment of morbid obesity in low-income adolescents: effects of parental self-monitoring. Obes Res 2005;13(9):1527–9.

88. Herman CP, Ostovich J, Polivy J. Effects of attentional focus on subjective hunger ratings. Appetite 1999;33(2):181–93.
89. Rogers PJ, Smit HJ. Food craving and food "addiction": a critical review of the evidence from a biopsychosocial perspective. Pharmacol Biochem Behav 2000;66(1):3–14.
90. Wright LB, Gregoski MJ, Tingen MS, et al. Impact of stress reduction interventions on hostility and ambulatory systolic blood pressure in African American adolescents. J Black Psychol 2011;37(2):210–33.
91. Edwards M, Adams EM, Waldo M, et al. Effects of mindfulness group of Latino adolescent students: Examining levels of perceived stress, mindfulness, self-compassion, and psychological symptoms. J Specialists Group Work 2014; 39(2):145–63.
92. Barnes VA, Treiber FA, Davis H, et al. Central Adiposity and Hemodynamic Functioning at Rest and During Stress in Adolescents. Inter J of Obes 1998;29(6): 997–1003.
93. Roemmich JN, Lambiase MJ, Lobarinas C, et al. Interactive effects of dietary restraint and adiposity on stress-induced eating and the food choice of children. Eat Beh 2011;12:309–12.
94. Verdejo-Garcia A, Moreno-Padilla M, Garcia-Rios MC, et al. Social stress increases cortisol and hampers attention in adolescents with excess weight. PLOS ONE 2015;10(4):1–2.
95. Smith BW, Shelley BM, Leahigh L, et al. A preliminary study of effects of a modified mindfulness intervention on binge eating. J of Evidence-Based Complementary and Alternative Medicine 2006;11(3):133–43.

Behavioral Economic Factors Related to Pediatric Obesity

Angela J. Jacques-Tiura, PhD[a],*, Mark K. Greenwald, PhD[b,c]

KEYWORDS

- Obesity • Pediatric • Behavioral economics • Incentives • Food reinforcement
- Demand • Energy intake • Physical activity

KEY POINTS

- Behavioral economics (BE) offers pathways for interventions to increase physical activity and healthier food intake and decrease sedentary behavior and unhealthy food consumption.
- BE suggests that pediatric clinicians should take careful behavioral histories, focused on the child's "marketplace" of food and activity options, to "nudge" behavior change.
- Clinicians and families must agree on the specific behaviors and time frame to be targeted for change, with the recognition that smaller, sustainable steps are more likely to be completed than more ambitious goals.

INTRODUCTION

Pediatric overweight and obesity are highly prevalent: about 32% of American children and adolescents are overweight (sex- and age-specific body mass index [BMI] 85th–95th percentile) or obese (BMI $\geq$ 95th percentile).[1] Although treatments have produced some improvements,[2] innovative nonmedication approaches are needed to curb this trend. Behavioral economics (BE) offers pathways for

Disclosures: This work was funded by Wayne State University Office of the Vice President for Research (Wayne State University Diabetes and Obesity Team Science), National Institutes of Health grants 2R01DA015462 and U01HL097889, Helene Lyckaki/Joe Young, Sr. Funds (State of Michigan), Detroit Wayne Mental Health Authority.
[a] Department of Family Medicine and Public Health Sciences, School of Medicine, iBio – Behavioral Health, Wayne State University, 6135 Woodward, H206, Detroit, MI 48202, USA; [b] Department of Psychiatry and Behavioral Neurosciences, School of Medicine, iBio –Behavioral Health, Wayne State University, Tolan Park Medical Building, 3901 Chrysler Service Drive, Suite 2A, Detroit, MI 48201, USA; [c] Department of Pharmacy Practice, Eugene Applebaum College of Pharmacy & Health Sciences, iBio –Behavioral Health, Wayne State University, Tolan Park Medical Building, 3901 Chrysler Service Drive, Suite 2A, Detroit, MI 48201, USA
* Corresponding author.
E-mail address: atiura@med.wayne.edu

interventions to increase physical activity (PA) and healthier food intake and decrease sedentary behavior and unhealthy food consumption. BE suggests that food and activity choices are governed by costs, available alternatives, and reinforcement. This article reviews basic and translational research using a BE framework with overweight or obese children up to age 18. We address BE concepts and methods, and discuss developmental issues, the continuum of BE approaches, findings of studies focused on increasing the cost of unwanted behaviors (ie, energy-dense food intake and sedentary behavior) and decreasing the cost of desired behaviors (ie, healthy food intake and PA), and our team's recent work using BE approaches with adolescents.

WHAT IS A BEHAVIORAL ECONOMIC APPROACH?

BE posits that reinforcers, available alternatives, and costs govern choices.[3] Holding other factors constant, individuals engage in behaviors that are highly reinforcing or have minimal suitable alternatives and lower costs (in money, time, or effort). **Box 1** includes key terms. For example, using a BE approach, interventionists may try to increase healthy eating by:

- Increasing the reinforcing properties of healthful foods (eg, touting the full flavors);
- Changing food environments to stock more healthful options than unhealthy options; and
- Lowering the cost of more healthful foods.

HOW MAY A BEHAVIORAL ECONOMIC APPROACH COMPLEMENT OTHER TREATMENT APPROACHES?

Because the BE approach focuses on changing environmental factors or reinforcers to change food- and PA-related behaviors, the BE approach is compatible with most currently available behavioral treatment approaches (eg, family-based lifestyle behavioral interventions), and could complement medication-assisted treatments once those come to fruition for pediatric obesity treatment. We emphasize that BE approaches should not be implemented in isolation but, rather, integrated with other viable strategies as part of multimodal, multilevel interventions.[4]

On the other hand, the BE approach, which relies on environmental sources of reinforcement to promote healthier outcomes (eg, weight loss), could potentially conflict with those cognitive–behavioral interventions that emphasize the importance of patients' internal motivation for behavior change (self-determination). Notably, there has been debate regarding this issue of exogenous versus endogenous locus of motivation elsewhere; namely, it has been hypothesized that external incentives could undermine a patient's internal motivation for behavior change. However, data supporting this conclusion are mixed[5–7]; rather than opposite ends of the motivation spectrum, intrinsic and extrinsic motivation seem to exist more independently than earlier thought.[8–10] A recent review of treatments for cannabis dependence demonstrated that long-term follow-up results from interventions combining contingency management (ie, giving vouchers for abstinence) and cognitive–behavioral therapy were better than for those using just 1 form of treatment,[11] suggesting that interventions targeting both intrinsic and extrinsic forms of motivation to change can be efficacious.

Compatibility of BE-based interventions with other treatment approaches partly depends on which outcomes are being targeted. Key questions in BE studies involve

Box 1
Definitions of key behavioral economic terms

Term	Definition
Behavioral economics (BE)	Interdisciplinary field at the intersection of economics and psychology, involving the analysis of purchasing/consumption of goods (eg, energy-dense food) in relation to constraints such as availability and price of a good and of competing goods (eg, nutritious foods) or activities (eg, physical activity). This field espouses that individuals do not always make rational decisions (unlike assumptions of classical economic theory that rely on "cold" calculation of utilities), potentially improving the predictive validity (translational value) of empirical studies.
Cross-price elasticity	Refers to how distinct reinforcers (eg, 2 different foods, or food vs nonfood item) interact in relation to their purchasing/consumption. The rate of change in consumption of a second good (at a constant UP) relative to change in UP of a first good. When UP increases in the first good result in less consumption, demand for the second good can increase (*substitute*), decrease (*complement*), or not change (*independent*). *Thought experiment*: consider situations in which these activities could serve as substitutes or complements: socializing, exercising, watching television, listening to music, eating an apple, and eating pie a la mode.
DD (also intertemporal discounting)	The DD procedure involves choices between an immediately consumable reinforcer of smaller value (eg, 1 candy bar now) and a deferred reinforcer of larger value (eg, 10 candy bars 1 week later), or choices between an consumable reinforcer now (eg, high-fat food) and a delayed punisher that could be mildly averse and briefly delayed (eg, gastrointestinal upset) or more delayed and more negative (eg, obesity, hypertension). When a subject prefers the smaller sooner option to the larger later option, s/he engages in steeper discounting of the delayed reward (exhibits less self-control).
Demand intensity	Amount of a good purchased/consumed at a very low (or free) unit price, that is without significant constraint. This amount corresponds to the *y*-intercept of the demand function.
Nudge	Implemented when evidence suggests individuals are making poor health (or other) decisions, a nudge is a programmed change in the person's environment to promote behavior that favors the individual's best interest. *Example*: Using a default 'opt-out' vs 'opt-in' for healthier choices.
Own-price elasticity	Measured in a specific context, the rate of change in consumption of a good relative to changes in its UP. Elasticity is not a fixed characteristic of a good (eg, physical activity or living in an environment with greater availability of healthy foods may increase price elasticity of some unhealthy foods). A good has *inelastic* demand when increases in its UP result in less-than-proportional decreases in consumption (ie, demand is relatively price-insensitive). A good has *elastic* demand when increases in its UP result in greater-than-proportional decreases in consumption (ie, demand is highly price-sensitive).
RRV	Goods are often available and can be purchased/consumed in competition with one another (ie, market conditions). RRV reflects the degree to which 1 good (eg, pizza slices) is purchased/consumed more than other concurrently available goods (eg, low-fat, low-calorie salad). RRV is not a fixed parameter of any good, and progressive increases in food RRV characterize obesigenic behavior.
UP	A ratio score that reflects the "cost" of a good (numerator) relative to the "benefit" or unit amount (eg, caloric, fat, sugar, or salt content of a single serving) of the good (denominator). "Cost" can include (but is not limited to) money price, or time/amount of responding (effort), required to purchase or consume a specified unit amount of a good.

Abbreviations: DD, delay discounting; RRV, relative reinforcing value; UP, unit price.

which behavior(s) will be reinforced, whether the behavior will be price sensitive (elastic), and how other available reinforcers will compete for control of behavior. The specific approach depends on the proposed mechanism of action in relation to the desired outcome, for example, increased healthy (or decreased unhealthy) food intake, increased PA (or decreased sedentary activities), increased energy expenditure (or decreased energy intake), or perhaps weight loss that is more distally mediated by the aforementioned factors.

In the case of increasing healthy nutrient intake, the BE approach presumes that greater availability and price-lowering manipulations will drive demand higher and, indirectly, could increase demand elasticity for unhealthy food. Conversely, if decreasing unhealthy nutrient intake is the focus, this presumes that demand for punished nutrient intake will become more price elastic and, indirectly, could result in more inelastic demand for healthy food. Similar BE substitutive relationships can be illustrated with regard to targeting behaviors associated with energy expenditure. Thus, when reinforcing PA one may observe a collateral reduction in sedentary activity, or when punishing a sedentary activity, one may observe an increase in PA. Both types of effects have been experimentally demonstrated in obese children.[12]

As noted, targeting more than 1 behavioral outcome (multimodal intervention) may be advantageous, but involves more complex mechanisms. A classic example is targeting both increased healthy nutrient intake and PA, which presumes these behaviors are compatible or, in BE terms, complementary. Increased PA might (aside from its acute anorectic effect) increase overall food consumption without regard to type of nutrient intake; thus, an intervention that seeks to increase desirable macronutrient consumption would be needed to narrow postexercise food intake. Consequently, a significant challenge of multimodal interventions will involve determining which reinforcers can serve as economic complements, so that desired outcomes are synergistically enhanced and undesired outcomes synergistically suppressed. Failure to consider these issues could result in 2 interventions that, although mildly effective in isolation, cancel each other's effects.

At the individual level, BE interventions can be used to decrease undesirable activities such as sedentary behavior (**Tables 1–3**). At the interpersonal level, BE approaches can be used to promote immersion of the individual in peer social networks that engage in PA and meaningfully interpersonal interactions, and/or discouraging sedentary behavior and unhealthy food intake.[13] It noteworthy that PA and sedentary behaviors, or eating healthy foods and avoiding unhealthy foods, are not necessarily substitute activities; rather, an inverse behavioral relationship must be demonstrated empirically in specific contexts when one manipulates one but not the other.[14,15]

Likewise, BE interventions can be targeted at the family level, for example, reinforcing behaviors of the caregiver (eg, purchasing predominantly healthy foods at the grocery store, restricting electronic media until after the child has exercised for 15 minutes) and the child (eg, eating enough fruits and vegetables, exercising 3 times weekly for 30 minutes each time). At the community level, BE approaches may be implemented within schools, afterschool centers, workplace cafeterias, or other centers in which food and activity choices are presented. Although many organizations may try an education approach, evidence suggests education alone may not improve behavior; on the other hand, pairing education with a reinforcer can increase healthier food choices.[19] Many of these are seen as "nudge" approaches,[44] in which consumers' choices are limited or restricted in some way to increase selection of healthier options.

CONTINUUM OF BEHAVIORAL ECONOMIC APPROACHES
Public Policy Stance

The Institute of Medicine's obesity prevention report[45] proposed a broad set of interventions to address obesity including child-focused measures such as positioning schools to function, in effect, as health centers (eg, promoting PA, banning high-sugar drinks). However, Marlow and Abdukadirov[46] have questioned this approach, noting that some regulatory interventions (eg, labeling/disclosure of nutrient content, taxing junk food) do not have reliable supporting data. They observe from the alcohol and tobacco literature that taxation approaches are not "one size fits all"; rather they tend to be more effective for individuals with less severe consumption problems (whose intake is price elastic) than those with greater problems (whose intake is price inelastic). These authors contend taxation will not be particularly effective for modifying unhealthy food intake among the real population of interest, obese individuals. They also argue that top-down regulatory policies, which are rational in their design, may not shift individual's food intake behaviors that are habit based (ie, irrational). Consistent with this hypothesis, Best and colleagues[30] found that children observed to have greater food relative reinforcing value (RRV) and who steeply discounted future food rewards at treatment baseline were less sensitive to an intervention that increased healthier food options in their natural environments.

Third-party Payers

Organizations that shoulder the economic burden from the consequences of unhealthy eating (eg, employers, insurers) have been paying attention to BE insights. From an actuarial perspective, the health benefits of interventions more readily accrue to individuals with less severe problems. Nonetheless, evidence from health incentive plans indicates it is possible to "nudge" employees' behavior through small, frequent payments—delivered outside of paychecks to increase their salience—for low-threshold, repeated healthy behaviors.[44]

Increasing the Availability of Healthy Foods

Particularly in urban and low-income settings, there is a critical need to reengineer the food environment to enable consumers (caregivers and children) to purchase and consume healthier foods. Many urban contexts suffer from being "food deserts," that is, there is a lack of ready access to healthy options that is dominated by unhealthy options. To remediate this problem, locally coordinated action is needed to reset the default options of the food economy, that is, to make healthy foods, rather than unhealthy foods, the salient market feature.[47] Community representatives (eg, legislators, philanthropists, business owners, religious organizations, educational institutions, and families) must work together to determine the best native solutions for investing in building and operating food markets. But, ideally, healthy food options should be located proximal to population centers and at the epicenter of community activities, thereby providing the opportunity to bring more people into greater contact with healthier food options. At the same time, we recognize that resetting default marketplace options is difficult and, even when this condition is met, this will not be sufficient for individuals' behavior change. For instance, it is equally necessary to increase the availability and salience of these healthy foods within the home environment. After purchasing foods, caregivers must monitor eating behaviors in the home environment. Taking a cue from the substance abuse literature again, parental monitoring is an effective preventive strategy for unwanted behaviors.

Table 1
Research studies aiming to increase healthy food (or decrease unhealthy food) choices and consumption

Authors	Population	Type of Study	Manipulation	Conclusion
Cravener et al,[16] 2015	24 3–5 y/o who consume <2 servings of vegetables/day and at least 1 parent with BMI ≥25; 8% minorities	Experimental, 4 wk RCT with 2 wk intervention period	Random assignment to treatment (families provided vegetables with favorite cartoon character and stickers as default choice for meals and snacks, granola bar available after 5-min wait) or control (generic packages of vegetables and granola bars)	Prekindergarten children's vegetable intake may be increased if vegetables are presented as default choice and paired with cartoon reinforcers.
Epstein et al,[17] study 1	35 8–12 y/o with BMI ≥ 85th percentile enrolled in FBT; average SES is upper middle class	Experimental and longitudinal	Random assignment to traditional FBT for weight loss or FBT + reinforcement for engaging in behavioral alternatives to eating	OW/obese preadolescents reinforced for weight loss engaged more in noneating activities than children in traditional FBT, but the increase was not related to weight changes.
Epstein et al,[17] study 2	13 8–12 y/o with BMI ≥ 85th percentile, average consumption of 2 snacks/day; 30% minorities	Experimental, within subjects	6 wk – 2 wk baseline, 2 wk enriched (kids given alternative activities to complete), 2 wk second baseline (enriched and second baseline counterbalanced)	OW/obese preadolescents spent more time in alternatives to screen and eating time, but that time did not translate to health outcomes.
Hanks et al,[18] 2012	Public high school students	Field study within high school; means from 2 days before and after manipulation compared	1 of 2 convenience lunch lines stocked only with healthier options for 8 wk after control "normal" 8 wk	If adolescents are given easy healthier options, they will take them (nudge effect).

Study	Sample	Design	Conditions	Findings
List & Samek,[19] 2015	1,614 children 7–18 y/o attending one of 24 "Kids Cafes" after-school programs in low-income areas of Chicago (most kids eligible for free or reduced price lunch program)	Experimental field study – sites randomized to dessert treatment condition with food choices recorded during extended baseline and treatment periods	Sites randomly assigned to no treatment, gain (child gets a prize if choose and eat fruit) short condition, loss (child given prize before dessert choice, if choose cookie or do not eat fruit choice, forfeit prize) long and short conditions, education long and short conditions, or education + loss long and short conditions	Incentives and educational messages paired with incentives, can increase choice and consumption of fruit over cookies whereas educational messages alone do not increase fruit consumption or choice.
Looney & Raynor,[20] 2012	80 4–9 y/o with BMI ≥ 85th–<95th percentile (OW) or ≥ 95th percentile (obese) and not meeting at least dietary or PA recommendation; <32% minority	Experimental, 6 mo family-based weight loss RCT	Random assignment to growth (increased growth monitoring to families), decrease (decrease snack food and sugar sweetened beverage consumption), or increase (increase fruit and vegetable and low-fat dairy intake)	Changes in fruit and vegetable and snack food were unrelated in these OW/obese children. Fruit and vegetable changes were unrelated to energy intake changes; reducing snack food led to reduction in energy intake.

Abbreviations: BMI, body mass index; FBT, family-based weight loss treatment; OW, overweight; PA, physical activity; RCT, randomized, controlled trial; SES, socioeconomic status.

Table 2
Research studies aiming to increase PA (or decrease sedentary activity) choices and consumption

Authors	Population	Type of Study	Manipulation	Conclusion
Epstein et al,[21] 2002 (subset of Epstein et al,[15] 2005)	13 8–12 y/o children; BMI < 95th percentile; 15–25 h/week sedentary activities; no systematic changes in factors related to energy intake/expenditure; average SES is upper middle class	Experimental within-subject crossover: baseline, increase, and decrease sedentary activity periods of 3 wk each	Increase and decrease sedentary behaviors as assigned; monetary incentives for appropriately changing sedentary activity levels	Among nonobese preadolescents, increasing sedentary behavior is related to greater kcal intake and less PA, leading to positive energy balance.
Epstein et al,[22] 2004	63 8–12 y/o BMI > 85th percentile; 10% minorities	Experimental 6 mo RCT to improve diet and PA, follow-up data collected at 6 and 12 mo	Random assignment to sedentary group (reinforced for time not spent sedentary activities) or stimulus control (reinforced for recording sedentary behaviors but not behavior change, instructed to change environment regarding sedentary activities)	Substituting PA for sedentary activity and complementing reduced snack foods with reduced sedentary activity can both produce weight loss, increased PA, and decreased sedentary activity time in these OW/obese preadolescents.
Epstein et al,[14] 2006 (further analysis of Epstein et al,[15] 2005)	58 8–16 y/o who report 15–25 h/week of screen time; average SES is upper middle class	Experimental within-subject crossover: baseline, increase, and decrease sedentary activity periods of 3 wk each. Related behavior to GIS coding.	Increase and decrease targeted sedentary behaviors (TV, video games, recreational computer use) as assigned; monetary incentives for changing sedentary activity levels.	Built environment matters – having a large park nearby led to increased PA and time in MVPA while sedentary behaviors were reduced.
Epstein et al,[15] 2005	58 8–16 y/o who report 15–25 h/week of screen time; 12% minorities	Experimental within-subject crossover: baseline, increase, and decrease sedentary activity periods of 3 wk each	Increase and decrease targeted sedentary behaviors (TV, video games, recreational computer use) as assigned; monetary incentives for appropriately changing sedentary activity levels	Sedentary and PA behaviors are largely substitutive; higher BMI kids more likely to decrease PA when sedentary behaviors increased; whereas children with lower general levels of PA were more likely to show greater increases in PA when sedentary activity decreased.

Study	Population	Design	Methods	Findings
Epstein et al,[23] 2005 (subset of Epstein et al,[15] 2005)	16 12–16 y/o with BMI < 95th percentile and report 15–25 h/week of screen time; average SES is upper middle class	Experimental within-subject crossover: baseline, increase, and decrease sedentary activity periods of 3 wk each	Increase and decrease targeted sedentary behaviors (TV, video games, recreational computer use) as assigned; monetary incentives for appropriately changing sedentary activity levels	Among nonobese adolescents, when targeted sedentary behaviors decrease, PA can increase and energy intake can decrease.
Epstein et al,[24] 2004	30 nonobese 8–12 y/o; 23% minorities	Experimental in laboratory random assignment of (1) access to all 4 PA and sedentary activities; (2) all 4 PA and least favorite sedentary activity; or (3) all 4 PA and favorite sedentary activity	RRV-PA vs sedentary assessed by computer task and questionnaire. In computer task, PA schedule remained at VR2; sedentary schedule increased from VR2 to VR32 over trials. Subjects asked whether willing to perform 20 button presses for 10 min of PA or 10 min of sedentary; then increasing number of button presses for sedentary	When constraining sedentary activity options to one less preferred, children engage less in sedentary option and more in PA; but challenging to substitute PA for sedentary activity when sedentary is highly valued and sedentary options are available.
Epstein et al,[12] 1995	27 obese 8–12 y/o	In laboratory experimental: group × type of activity × day	Random assignment to activity group (reinforced for time spent in active options), sedentary group (reinforced for time not spent in 2 preferred sedentary activities), or control. Over 5 daily sessions, given access to 4 active and 4 sedentary for 45 min	Reducing access (either via reinforcing activity or nonengagement) can increase time spent in active activities among obese children.

(continued on next page)

Table 2
(continued)

Authors	Population	Type of Study	Manipulation	Conclusion
Epstein et al,[25] exp 1	18 kids, M age = 10.5 y/o, lean (<20% over average weight), moderately obese (20%-80% over average weight), very obese (>80% over average weight). Some obese kids starting FBT for weight loss	In laboratory	Computer game with unchanging variable ratio reinforcement of vigorous activity (bike riding) and ascending or descending variable ratio reinforcement for sedentary activity (watching videos)	When sedentary activities have high costs, lean and some obese children will choose PA; some more obese children will work for sedentary regardless of cost.
Epstein et al,[25] exp 2	23 obese kids, M age = 10.1 y/o (20%–100% OW)	In laboratory	Computer game with unchanging VR reinforcement of highly liked or disliked vigorous activity and ascending or descending VR reinforcement for sedentary activity (watching videos)	When costs are the same, obese children choose sedentary activities; but when costs increase, children may switch to vigorous activity.
Epstein et al,[26] 1995	61 obese 8–12 y/o, between 20% and 100% OW but neither parent >100% OW; 4% minorities	Experimental 4 mo RCT to improve diet and PA	Randomly assigned to reinforcing decreased sedentary activity, reinforcing increased PA, or reinforcing both	Reinforcement for reducing sedentary activity produce better weight outcomes than reinforcing increased PA in these obese preadolescents.

Study	Sample	Design	Method	Findings
Goldfield et al,[27] 2000	34 8-12 y/o children with BMI ≥ 85th percentile, enrolled in family-based pediatric obesity treatment study; average SES is upper middle class	Experimental in laboratory, random assignment to 1 of 3 groups	Requirement of accumulating 1,500 (or 750) pedometer counts of PA in 20 min to earn 10 min of TV activity vs control (access to PA and TV activity for 30 min)	OW/obese children engage in more PA if reinforced with preferred sedentary activities.
Goldfield et al,[28] 2006	30 8-12 y/o with BMI ≥ 85th percentile who watch ≥15 h TV/week and engage in <30 min MVPA/day and have parent willing to enforce study contingencies	8 wk RCT	Kids randomly assigned to open-loop feedback + reinforcement (accumulating 400 PA counts earns the kid 1 h of TV viewing) or just open-loop feedback (wear accelerometer but no activity restrictions)	OW/obese children exhibit health improvements (eg, decrease weight, BMI, fat intake, calories from snacks, and snack patterns) and increase PA time if reinforced.
Salvy et al,[29] 2009	88 12-14 y/o; 19% minorities	Experimental: 2 (weight: ≥ or < 85th percentile) × 2 (gender) × 2 (social context: alone vs friend or peer) mixed design	2 sessions: (1) RRV of biking alone vs playing video games alone, (2) RRV of biking with a friend or with a peer (randomly assigned)	Presence of a friend or unfamiliar peer can increase motivation (RRV) to engage in PA (bike riding) and to bike longer, especially for OW children.

Abbreviations: BMI, body mass index; FBT, family-based weight loss treatment; MVPA, moderate-to-vigorous physical activity; OW, overweight; PA, physical activity; RCT, randomized, controlled trial; RRV, relative reinforcing value; SES, socioeconomic status; VR, variable ratio.

Table 3
Other research studies related to weight loss, intake, or activity using a BE approach

Authors	Population	Type of Study	Manipulation	Conclusion
Best et al,[30] 2012	241 OW (BMI ≥ 85th percentile) 7–12 y/o with ≥1 parent with BMI ≥25, FBT treatment; 35% minorities	Prospective, with BE factors treated as baseline predictors of weight loss	Assessed RRV-food (HED), RRV-money, DD-money, DD-food, environmental enrichment (availability of alternatives)	Pretreatment individual differences matter. Weight loss less for children who were more impulsive with money reward, and for food-impulsive children highly reinforced by food. Having better alternatives in home environment helped children less reinforced by food lose more weight.
Epstein et al,[31] 2007	35 8–12 y/o (17 non-OW with BMI < 85th percentile; 18 OW with BMI > 95th percentile); 26% minority	In laboratory	Computer choice task (RRV) for active and sedentary alternatives for dancing and bike riding, reinforcement schedule increased from VR8 to VR128	Children were more motivated to play an interactive dance video game but not for an interactive (vs other form) bike video game.
Epstein et al,[32] 2015	198 8–12 y/o; BMI percentile between 50th and 85th or <50th with parent BMI ≥ 25; 31% minority	In laboratory	Questionnaire version of RRV of favorite sweet, savory, and salty foods vs access to magazines and word games	Sweet foods most reinforcing among non-OW children, but may be overall RRV-food related to higher energy intake.
Epstein et al,[33] 2006 (subset of Epstein et al,[15] 2005)	10 10–12 y/o and their mothers; 20% African American	In laboratory	Food choice task in which subjects were given $5 in $0.25 tokens to spend on snack or fruit/vegetable. Across trials, 1 food remained $1 and others varied from $0.50 to $2.50	Mothers' purchasing of healthy and unhealthy foods related to their child's purchasing; for both food types as cost increased, purchasing decreased.

Study	Sample	Setting	Method	Findings
Epstein et al,[34] 2008	50 8–12 y/o with BMI $\geq$ 85th percentile and parents; 30% minorities	In laboratory	Paper questionnaire assessing RRV-food and money (vs other) and computer-based DD task	RRV-food is related in kids and their parents. DD depends on magnitude of immediate reward but kids were more impulsive than parents. Parents' and kids' DD not related.
Epstein et al,[35] study 1	32 10–12 y/o; 35% minority	In laboratory	Food choice task in which subjects were given $5 in $0.25 tokens to spend on snack or fruit/vegetable. Across trials, 1 food remained $1 and others varied from $0.50 to $2.50	Youths' food purchasing depended on its price and price of alternative, but substitution did not occur.
Epstein et al,[35] study 2	20 10–14 y/o; 25% minorities	In laboratory	Food choice task in which subjects given $1, $3, or $5 in imitation coins to spend on snack or fruit/vegetable. Across trials, 1 food set remained at market value; 1 set varied from 50% below to 50% above market value	Findings support own-price elasticity. Substitution of alternatives depended on amount of money available to spend (income). Substitution only occurred with low income.
Epstein et al,[36] 1999	32 6–11 y/o, recruited for studies (1) to prevent childhood obesity in nonobese kids with obese parents, or (2) to modify food intake in obese kids; 6% minority	In laboratory, relating computer-assessed RRV of PA and sedentary activities with 4 days of naturalistic activity data	Computer game to assess RRV of concurrently available sedentary activities (Nintendo game, videos, reading, coloring) or PA (bicycle ergometer or stepper). PA reinforced on VR2 schedule, whereas sedentary schedule increased from VR2 to VR16 across games	The more reinforcing children find PA, the more physically active they are. Multiple shorter PA sessions may be more reinforcing than fewer longer sessions.

(continued on next page)

Table 3
(continued)

Authors	Population	Type of Study	Manipulation	Conclusion
Epstein et al,[37] 2014	130 nonobese (BMI < 95th percentile) adolescents (M age = 15.2 y); 21% minorities	In laboratory, relating computer-assessed RRV of money and favorite snack food with BMI change over 2 y	Computer choice task (RRV) for money and favorite snack food	Higher BMI z score associated with finding snack foods more reinforcing (and having more obese parents).
Hill et al,[38] 2009	316 7–9 y/o (baseline) enrolled in 1 of 5 schools in London, UK; 54% non-white	Observational, longitudinal design	Questionnaire version of RRV of cookies vs stickers on PR schedule	Children who find food more reinforcing than stickers gain more weight over 1 year
Kong et al,[39] study 1	27 9.0–18.6 mo olds; weight-for-length z scores ranged from −1.50 to 2.55; 22% minority; 64% family income >$50k	In laboratory	Computer mouse to work for favorite food or Baby Einstein video clips on sequential, independent PR schedule	Infants and toddlers at risk for obesity demonstrated greater food than video reinforcement, and low reinforcement levels for the video.
Kong et al,[39] study 2	30 8.9–17.8 mo olds; weight-for-length z scores ranged from −1.03 to 2.65; 11% minority; 53% family income >$50k	In laboratory	Computer mouse to work for favorite food or bubbles play time on sequential, independent PR schedule	Infants and toddlers at risk for obesity demonstrated greater food than video reinforcement, and low reinforcement levels for the bubbles activity.
Penko & Barkley,[40] 2010	24 8–12 y/o; 11 lean (BMI < 85th percentile) and 13 OW/obese (BMI ≥ 85th percentile)	In laboratory	Computer mouse to work for Wii vs sedentary video boxing game access on independent PR schedule	Lean children find active games more reinforcing than sedentary games (and more so than OW children) but OW children found them equally reinforcing (and sedentary game more reinforcing than for lean children).

Study	Sample	Setting	Task	Findings
Rollins et al,[41] 2014	33 3–5 y/o; BMI percentiles ranged from 3.2 to 95.7; 24% not White; 64% of families' income >$80k	Conducted at preschools	Computer station to work for Scooby Doo and Sponge Bob graham crackers on independent, concurrent PR schedule	Preschoolers are willing to work for snacks. Children with higher BMI and reward sensitivity levels worked faster to access the snacks, and faster (and more) responding corresponded with snack consumption in a separate task
Salvy et al,[42] 2012	103 adolescents (M age = 13.6 y); 21% minorities	In laboratory, relating RRV-food and social interaction with ostracism manipulation, sedentary activity tasks, eating, conversing with peer	Computer choice task (RRV) for social interaction time and favorite snack food	Ostracized adolescents may have higher motivation for obtaining favorite snack foods.
Temple et al,[43] Exp 1	45 8–12 y/o (20 with BMI ≥ 90th percentile; 25 with BMI < 75th percentile); 27% minorities	In laboratory	Computer station to work for pizza or nonfood alternative on VR schedule	OW children find food (pizza) more reinforcing (willing to work harder to get it), and consume more of it than non-OW children
Temple et al,[43] Exp 2	45 8–12 y/o (20 with BMI ≥ 85th percentile; 25 with BMI < 85th percentile); 23% minorities	In laboratory	Computer station to work for liked snack food (chips, Skittles, M&M's) or nonfood alternative on VR schedule	OW children find food (snacks) more reinforcing/are willing to work harder to get it than to get sedentary activities, and consume more of it than non-OW children

Abbreviations: BE, behavioral economic; BMI, body mass index; DD, delay discounting; FBT, family-based weight loss treatment; HED, high energy dense; OW, overweight; PA, physical activity; PR, progressive ratio; RRV, relative reinforcing value; SES, socioeconomic status; VR, variable ratio.

Behavioral Commitment

At an organizational level, considerable evidence has accrued to indicate that health behaviors can be promoted through default opt-out plans than default opt-in plans. This observation could be owing to the 'endowment effect' (overattachment to existing reinforcers or lifestyle) and/or to the effort required to switch (representing a cost or price).

At the individual level, having people make written plans can motivate behavior change. The mechanism of this behavioral effect could stem from delay discounting: If the person can envision the temporal horizon for completing a concrete behavior (which is being examined by use of "episodic future thinking" interventions),[48–52] it becomes more salient than alternatives. Another possible explanation is that the written plan may—particularly in a social context—solidify personal intention (a promissory note, of sorts) by decreasing the temptation to escape the commitment to avoid shame.

Developmental Considerations

BE-based research, specifically assessing RRV (of food, activity, or other commodities), has been conducted with infants as young as 9 months,[39] and with toddlers, preschoolers, young school-age children, and adolescents. Children across ages demonstrate individual differences in their level of reinforcement from food; a key factor to consider is how to assess RRV. Infants can learn to press buttons to get what they want, and older children can learn a variety of computer-based games or understand questionnaires. Younger children may be more amenable to increasing PA by decreasing sedentary activity.[14,36] Gender differences are not often found, but mixed results have been reported (girls biked more than boys in a video game experiment,[31] boys were more likely to substitute physical for sedentary activity,[14,22] and boys indicated stronger reinforcement from food).[39,41] Brain substrates underlying impulsivity and self-control mechanisms—mediated by frontal-cortical regions—are less well-developed in children and adolescents relative to adults, as evidenced in larger delay discounting for children.[34]

CURRENT STATE OF THE BASIC, TRANSLATIONAL, AND INTERVENTION LITERATURE ON BEHAVIORAL ECONOMICS–RELATED FACTORS IN PEDIATRIC OBESITY
Increasing Consumption of Healthy Foods

Table 1 describes 6 intervention studies focused on food intake, including both those studies that aim to increase consumption of healthy foods and studies that aim to decrease consumption of unhealthy foods. BE suggests that when the price (in money, time, or other costs) of healthy foods is lowered, children may increase consumption. Easing access in a high school cafeteria increased intake of healthier options and decreased consumption of less healthy options.[18] Incentives paired with healthy options can increase consumption in both preschoolers[16] and older children.[19] Healthy and unhealthy foods are not necessarily substitutes for one another, however. For example, among children randomized to decreasing their snack food consumption; increasing their fruit, vegetable, and low-fat dairy intake; or increased growth monitoring, fruit and vegetable intake increased during treatment but intake was unrelated to decreases in snack food intake or total energy intake.[20] Although snack food consumption did not decrease significantly, reductions were associated significantly with energy intake reductions. Further, reinforcing engagement in alternative activities to eating may increase such engagement overall, but such changes may not be enough to meaningfully affect weight.[17]

Taken together, research focused on increasing consumption of healthier foods suggests:

- Using incentives paired with healthy options;
- Altering default choices to healthier options; and
- Decreasing energy-dense food consumption rather than increasing healthier foods consumption to decrease energy consumption.

Increasing Physical Activity

Table 2 describes 13 basic research and intervention studies focused on increasing PA, including those studies reinforcing increased PA itself and those reinforcing not engaging in sedentary activities. The goal of providing incentives for exercise and social activity are based on the BE idea that these activities can compete with energy-dense food consumption and, thus, can function as economic substitutes. It has been noted that the RRV of PA may be greater when such activity occurs in multiple, short bouts rather than fewer, extended bouts.[36] This is tantamount to lowering the short-term unit price of PA and, from the perspective of delay discounting, making it more feasible in the present time. Several studies found that PA can substitute for sedentary activity among nonoboese[15,21–23,25] and sometimes among obese[12,25] children. Not surprisingly, substitution of PA for sedentary activity is more likely when the child is less reinforced by the sedentary activity.[24] Using time for sedentary activity as a reinforcer for engaging in PA may also encourage some obese children to increase their PA level[27] and improve health outcomes.[28] An early study demonstrated that reinforcing reducing time spent in sedentary activity may produce better weight outcomes among obese children than reinforcing increased time spent in PA, perhaps because the children had more autonomy with their time not spent sedentary. Overweight children may benefit from engaging in PA with other children, because the presence of another child can increase reinforcement from PA.

Taken together, research focused on increasing PA suggests that:

- Decreasing sedentary time may increase physically active time;
- Treating sedentary time as a reinforcer for physically active time may increase physically active time; and
- Engaging in PA with another child may increase reinforcement for overweight children.

Nudging

Health behaviors are difficult to initiate. The baseline conditions of a person's environment set a default behavior mode (status quo) that is hard to overcome. Thus, it may be necessary to breach that gap by resetting the baseline conditions (eg, where the caregiver shops for food, stocking a lunch line with tasty healthier options[18]). Likewise, health behaviors are also notoriously difficult to maintain, and the incentives used to sustain behavior changes may necessitate increasing the frequency of monitoring and reinforcement. In this regard, technology is a useful handmaiden of behavior change in the obesity prevention/treatment field because electronic messaging (eg, well-timed reminders to exercise or eat certain foods) can overcome limitations of traditional office-based interventions. More research is needed in the area of nudging.

Individual Differences as Mediators/Moderators of Behavioral Economics–Inspired Interventions

Table 3 describes 17 basic and translational research studies of factors that may moderate, mediate, or otherwise influence BE-guided intervention effects. As noted, incentive approaches may work better for individuals whose demand is less intense and/or price elastic.[30] Overweight and obese children typically find foods and sedentary activity more reinforcing, and PA less reinforcing, than lean children,[39–41,43] and increasing weight is associated with higher reinforcement from snack foods.[37,38] Ostracized adolescents (those excluded from the group) may find energy-dense food more reinforcing,[42] suggesting that more engagement with other children may be beneficial for reinforcement from food and PA. Impulsivity (ie, failure of self-control), mediated by frontal-cortical brain regions, is correlated with greater energy-dense food intake, and needs to be considered as a constraint on behavior change.[30] Thus, interventions must weigh incentive value (positive reinforcement of healthy, or punishment of unhealthy, food Intake) against underlying impulsive tendencies of the individual (potentially associated with younger age of the child) that will tend to undermine these efforts.

Another individual difference characteristic that closely relates to BE-inspired tactics is income level, which can moderate the food purchasing/consumption. Specifically, increases in income may ameliorate substitution of lower cost healthier options for more favored and more expensive less healthy options.[35] When income is constrained, substitution may occur if healthy choices have lower costs than unhealthy choices.[35] Children's healthy and unhealthy choices can be elastic.[35]

An additional factor to consider when evaluating the reinforcing value of food and activity is what exact commodities are being measured and compared. For example, lean children find an active video game (boxing) more reinforcing than the sedentary version, but overweight children found them equally reinforcing (although the lean and overweight children differed in how reinforcing each type was),[31] and dancing and bicycling riding are both physical activities, but motivation to engage in each vary, as did how to engage in them as video games.[40] Among lean children, the RRV of sweet foods was highest but the RRV of sweet, salty, and savory foods were all correlated and their combination was associated with energy intake.[32]

Taken together, other BE-guided research suggests that:

- Weight status, impulsivity, income, feelings of inclusion, and type of commodity may serve as moderators or mediators of intervention effects.

CURRENT AND FUTURE DIRECTIONS

Tables 1–3 demonstrate that the majority of BE-guided research is conducted with primarily White, upper middle class samples (with notable exceptions[19,30,35,38]). Our team is investigating the role of RRV in basic research and as a moderator of intervention treatment effects in African American adolescents. In our Sequential Multiple Assignment Randomized Trial (SMART),[53] African American adolescents (12–16 y/o) with obesity (BMI $\geq$ 95th percentile) completed 3 months of motivational interviewing plus skills building with their caregivers in their home or clinic (first randomization). Adolescents who did not lose at least 3% of their baseline body weight were re-randomized to complete 3 months of contingency management (reinforcement for weight loss) or additional skill building in their home. At baseline, we measured adolescents' RRV of a favorite snack food using a food purchase task questionnaire. Preliminary analyses indicate that adolescents' RRV interacted with treatment sequence to influence weight loss and reduction of symptoms of the metabolic syndrome. These findings highlight the need to assess individual differences in RRV at the start of treatment.[30]

In an ongoing laboratory study with a sample of African American adolescents and caregivers, we are determining whether caregiver food purchasing is related to their child's BMI (12–17 years old). Each caregiver completes a typical shopping trip for their household in a 'virtual grocery store' where each item is displayed with its picture, nutritional information, package size, and local price. Participants place items in their grocery cart and amount spent is displayed during shopping. We will compare caregivers' virtual shopping behavior with their recent real-world grocery receipts as a validation test of the experimental model. That this is a low-SES urban sample with relatively low access to traditional large grocery stores and frequent use of convenience and "corner stores" is a novel experience that could provide revealing information regarding food purchasing behaviors. This virtual grocery store model is expected to provide data relevant to food price-elasticity that may be useful in intervention studies and policy planning.

In this same project, we are determining whether adolescent BMI is related to food demand, particularly in relationship to a stressor. In 2 separate experimental sessions (stress [listening to crying babies] and neutral [listening to nature sounds] in randomized order), each adolescent can work for unit amounts of 2 foods on 11 independent choice trials: his or her preferred high-palatable food (1 Oreo or 5 Doritos per trial; determined at screening) or 1 baby carrot. In each 30-minute session, we vary food unit price by increasing the response requirement (number of mouse clicks) for each successive same-food choice on a progressive ratio schedule as in our recent work.[54] The adolescent can consume his or her earned food after each session, and we measure the amount and rate of consumption. We measure heart rate and saliva cortisol as a manipulation check on stress reactivity. Preliminary findings indicate that teens with higher (questionnaire-based) levels of food disinhibition and automaticity consume more snack food following the experimental stressor. Our future work will build on this project by expanding the menu ("mini-buffet" model) in the food choice task, and examining how engaging in PA of varying intensities before the food choice task affects biomarker, neurocognitive, and food-reinforced responding among African American adolescents with obesity.

SUMMARY/DISCUSSION

With regard to improving children's eating and activity behaviors, BE posits that reinforcers, available alternatives, and costs govern choices. The research reviewed here demonstrates that:

- Environmental factors powerfully affect choice and nudges may improve personal and population health;
- Food and activity reinforcement value varies across children (eg, owing to trait or other historical factors), age, and possibly gender;
- Higher pretreatment food and lower activity reinforcement may decrease the success of weight loss interventions for youth;
- Children may substitute PA for sedentary activity if reinforced; and
- More ethnically and financially diverse samples are needed.

Although the American Academy of Pediatrics has made recommendations to pediatric health care providers to promote family diets that are rich in fruits and vegetables, low in energy-dense products, balanced with greater engagement in PA and less engagement in sedentary activities,[55] there are feasibility challenges in how to communicate and achieve these goals. The BE framework suggests that pediatric clinicians should take careful behavioral histories (perhaps aided by staff with specialized behavioral training), focused on the child's "marketplace" of food and activity options (influenced at the person, caregiver/family, and school/community levels), to identify barriers (ie, opportunity costs of foregoing currently preferred activities for new ones) and incentives (eg, changing the default options, and milestone rewards) to "nudge" behavior change.[56] Clinicians and families must agree on the specific behaviors and time frame to be targeted for change, with recognition that smaller, sustainable steps are more likely to be completed (less delay discounting, lower price) than more ambitious goals.

REFERENCES

1. Ogden CL, Carroll MD, Kit BK, et al. Prevalence of childhood and adult obesity in the United States, 2011-2012. JAMA 2014;311(8):806–14.
2. Altman M, Wilfley DE. Evidence update on the treatment of overweight and obesity in children and adolescents. J Clin Child Adolesc Psychol 2015;44(4): 521–37.
3. Bickel WK, Vuchinich RE, editors. Reframing health behavior change with behavioral economics. Mahwah (NJ): Lawrence Erlbaum Associates; 2000.
4. Huang TT, Drewnowski A, Kumanyika SK, et al. A systems-oriented multilevel framework for addressing obesity in the 21st century. Prev Chronic Dis 2009; 6(3):A82.
5. Deci EL, Koestner R, Ryan RM. A meta-analytic review of experiments examining the effects of extrinsic rewards on intrinsic motivation. Psychol Bull 1999;125: 626–68.
6. Ledgerwood DM, Petry NM. Does contingency management affect motivation to change substance use? Drug Alcohol Depend 2006;83:65–72.
7. Ng JY, Ntoumanis N, Thørgersen-Ntoumani C, et al. Self-determination theory applied to health contexts: a meta-analysis. Perspect Psychol Sci 2012;7:325–40.
8. Gerhart B, Fang M. Pay, intrinsic motivation, extrinsic motivation, performance, and creativity in the workplace: revisiting long-held beliefs. Annu Rev Organ Psychol Organ Behav 2015;2:489–521.
9. Lepper MR, Corpus JH, Iyengar SS. Intrinsic and extrinsic motivational orientations in the classroom: age differences and academic correlates. J Educ Psychol 2005;97:184–96.
10. Naar-King S, Suarez M. Integrating motivational interviewing into your practice. In: Naar-King S, Suarez M, editors. Motivational interviewing with adolescents and young adults. New York: Guilford; 2011. p. 75–84.
11. Cooper K, Chatters R, Kaltenthaler E, et al. Psychological and psychosocial interventions for cannabis cessation in adults: a systematic review short report. Health Technol Assess 2015;19(56):1–130.
12. Epstein LH, Saelens BE, O'Brien JG. Effects of reinforcing increases in active behavior versus decreases in sedentary behavior for obese children. Int J Behav Med 1995;2(1):41–50.
13. Epstein LH, Wrotniak BH. Future directions for pediatric obesity treatment. Obesity (Silver Spring) 2010;18:S8–12.
14. Epstein LH, Raja S, Gold SS, et al. Reducing sedentary behavior: the relationship between park area and the physical activity of youth. Psychol Sci 2006;17:654–9.
15. Epstein LH, Roemmich JN, Paluch RA, et al. Physical activity as a substitute for sedentary behavior in youth. Ann Behav Med 2005;29(3):200–9.
16. Cravener TL, Schlechter H, Loeb KL, et al. Feeding strategies derived from behavioral economics and psychology can increase vegetable intake in children as part of a home-based intervention: results of a pilot study. J Acad Nutr Diet 2015;115:1798–807.

17. Epstein LH, Roemmich JN, Stein RI, et al. The challenge of identifying behavioral alternatives to food: clinic and field studies. Ann Behav Med 2005;30(3):201–9.
18. Hanks AS, Just DR, Smith LE, et al. Healthy convenience: nudging students toward healthier choices in the lunchroom. J Public Health (Oxf) 2012;34(3):370–6.
19. List JA, Samek AS. The behavioralist as nutritionist: leveraging behavioral economics to improve child food choice and consumption. J Health Econ 2015;39: 135–46.
20. Looney SM, Raynor HA. Are changes in consumption of "healthy" foods related to changes in consumption of "unhealthy" foods during pediatric obesity treatment? Int J Environ Res Public Health 2012;9(4):1368–78.
21. Epstein LH, Paluch RA, Consalvi A, et al. Effects of manipulating sedentary behavior on physical activity and food intake. J Pediatr 2002;140:334–9.
22. Epstein LH, Paluch RA, Kilanowski CK, et al. The effect of reinforcement or stimulus control to reduce sedentary behavior in the treatment of pediatric obesity. Health Psychol 2004;23:371–80.
23. Epstein LH, Roemmich JN, Paluch RA, et al. Influence of changes in sedentary behavior on energy and macronutrient intake in youth. Am J Clin Nutr 2005;81: 361–6.
24. Epstein LH, Roemmich JN, Saad FG, et al. The value of sedentary alternatives influences child physical activity choice. Int J Behav Med 2004;11:236–42.
25. Epstein LH, Smith JA, Vara LS, et al. Behavioral economic analysis of activity choice in obese children. Health Psychol 1991;10:311–6.
26. Epstein LH, Valoski AM, Vara LS, et al. Effects of decreasing sedentary behavior and increasing activity on weight change in obese children. Health Psychol 1995; 14:109–15.
27. Goldfield GS, Kalakanis LE, Ernst MM, et al. Open-loop feedback to increase physical activity in obese children. Int J Obes Relat Metab Disord 2000;24(7): 888–92.
28. Goldfield GS, Mallory R, Parker T, et al. Effects of open-loop feedback on physical activity and television viewing in overweight and obese children: a randomized, controlled trial. Pediatrics 2006;118(1):e157–166.
29. Salvy SJ, Roemmich JN, Bowker JC, et al. Effect of peers and friends on youth physical activity and motivation to be physically active. J Pediatr Psychol 2009; 34(2):217–25.
30. Best JR, Theim KR, Gredysa DM. Behavioral economic predictors of overweight children's weight loss. J Consult Clin Psychol 2012;80(6):1086–96.
31. Epstein LH, Beecher MD, Graf JL, et al. Choice of interactive dance and bicycle games in overweight and non-overweight youth. Ann Behav Med 2007;33(2): 124–31.
32. Epstein LH, Carr KA, Scheid JL, et al. Taste and food reinforcement in non-overweight youth. Appetite 2015;91:226–32.
33. Epstein LH, Dearing KK, Handley EA. Relationship of mother and child food purchases as a function of price: a pilot study. Appetite 2006;47:115–8.
34. Epstein LH, Dearing KK, Temple JL, et al. Food reinforcement and impulsivity in overweight children and their parents. Eat Behav 2008;9:319–27.
35. Epstein LH, Handley KA, Dearing KK, et al. Purchases of food in youth: influence of price and income. Psychol Sci 2006;17:82–9.
36. Epstein LH, Kilanowski CK, Consalvi AR, et al. Reinforcing value of physical activity as a determinant of child activity level. Health Psychol 1999;18:599–603.
37. Epstein LH, Yokum S, Feda DM, et al. Food reinforcement and parental obesity predict future weight gain in non-obese adolescents. Appetite 2014;82:138–42.

38. Hill C, Saxton J, Webber L, et al. The relative reinforcing value of food predicts weight gain in a longitudinal study of 7-10-y-old children. Am J Clin Nutr 2009; 90(2):276–81.
39. Kong KL, Feda D, Eiden R, et al. Origins of food reinforcement in infants. Am J Clin Nutr 2015;101(3):515–22.
40. Penko AL, Barkley JE. Motivation and physiologic responses of playing a physically interactive video game relative to a sedentary alternative in children. Ann Behav Med 2010;39(2):162–9.
41. Rollins BY, Loken E, Savage JS, et al. Measurement of food reinforcement in preschool children: associations with food intake, BMI, and reward sensitivity. Appetite 2014;72:21–7.
42. Salvy SJ, Bowker JC, Nitecki LA, et al. Effects of ostracism and social connection-related activities on adolescents' motivation to eat and energy intake. J Pediatr Psychol 2012;37(1):23–32.
43. Temple JL, Legierski CM, Giacomelli AM, et al. Overweight children find food more reinforcing and consume more energy than do nonoverweight children. Am J Clin Nutr 2008;87(5):1121–7.
44. Loewenstein G, Asch DA, Volpp KG. Behavioral economics holds potential to deliver better results for patients, insurers, and employers. Health Aff (Millwood) 2013;32(7):1244–50.
45. Institute of Medicine (IOM). Accelerating progress in obesity prevention: solving the weight of the nation. Washington, DC: The National Academies Press; 2012.
46. Marlow ML, Abdukadirov S. Can behavioral economics combat obesity? Regulation 2012;35(2):14–8.
47. Gittelsohn J, Lee K. Integrating educational, environmental, and behavioral economic strategies may improve the effectiveness of obesity interventions. Appl Econ Perspect Pol 2013;35(1):52–68.
48. O'Neill J, Daniel TO, Epstein LH. Episodic future thinking reduces eating in a food court. Eat Behav 2015;20:9–13.
49. Dassen FC, Jansen A, Nederkoorn C, et al. Focus on the future: episodic future thinking reduces discount rate and snacking. Appetite 2015;96:327–32.
50. Daniel TO, Said M, Stanton CM, et al. Episodic future thinking reduces delay discounting and energy intake in children. Eat Behav 2015;18:20–4.
51. Daniel TO, Stanton CM, Epstein LH. The future is now: reducing impulsivity and energy intake using episodic future thinking. Psychol Sci 2013;24(11):2339–42.
52. Daniel TO, Stanton CM, Epstein LH. The future is now: comparing the effect of episodic future thinking on impulsivity in lean and obese individuals. Appetite 2013;71:120–5.
53. Naar-King S, Ellis D, Idalski Carcone A, et al. Sequential multiple assignment randomized trial (SMART) to construct weight loss interventions for African American adolescents. J Clin Child Adolesc Psychol 2015;1–14 [Epub ahead of print].
54. Reslan S, Saules KK, Greenwald MK. Validating a behavioral economic approach to assess food demand: effects of body mass index, dietary restraint, and impulsivity. Appetite 2012;59:364–71.
55. Daniels SR, Hassink SG; Committee on Nutrition. The role of the pediatrician in primary prevention of obesity. Pediatrics 2015;136:e275–92.
56. Wilfley DE, Kass AE, Kolko RP. Counseling and behavior change in pediatric obesity. Pediatr Clin North Am 2011;58:1403–24.

Neurocognitive Processes and Pediatric Obesity Interventions

Review of Current Literature and Suggested Future Directions

Alison L. Miller, PhD

KEYWORDS

• Pediatric obesity • Executive functioning • Behavior change • Intervention

KEY POINTS

- Incorporating a focus on self-regulation as an underlying mechanism of health behavior change may lead to better health outcomes.
- Executive functioning (EF) is a central aspect of self-regulation, and EF skill deficits are associated with higher weight status and obesity-promoting risk factors in children.
- Different aspects of EF may be associated with obesity risk at different points in development.
- Behavioral techniques to enhance EF in children may provide a new tool for obesity prevention, particularly for children characterized by high sensitivity to food reward or social-contextual risks.

INTRODUCTION

Childhood obesity is a critical and ongoing public health problem, with almost 25% of children overweight by age 4 years and 35% by adolescence.[1] Once established, childhood obesity is difficult to treat and tracks into adulthood.[2] There is thus an urgent need to prevent and treat childhood obesity, but current prevention and treatment approaches focused on improving diet and physical activity patterns have had limited efficacy.[3] One reason for this may be a lack of focus on the basic mechanisms of behavior change,[4] specifically self-regulation processes that may shape whether recommended health behaviors are adopted. If enhancing self-regulation in childhood

Conflicts of Interest: The author has no commercial or financial conflicts of interest.
Funding: NIH 1UH2HD087979 to A.L. Miller.
Department of Health Behavior and Health Education, University of Michigan School of Public Health, 1415 Washington Heights, SPH I, Ann Arbor, MI 48109, USA
E-mail address: alimill@umich.edu

could improve health behaviors relevant for obesity prevention, this may lead to new intervention targets and, in turn, better long-term health outcomes.

Self-regulation occurs at many levels (cognitive, emotional, psychological, biological, behavioral) and concerns the ability to control thoughts, emotions, and actions to achieve a desired outcome or goal.[5–7] Self-regulation can shape health behaviors through multiple pathways. For example, the ability to delay an immediate desired behavioral reward (eg, eating a cookie) in favor of achieving a longer-term goal (eg, weight loss) is a central focus of most weight management approaches. Furthermore, having the cognitive capacity to plan ahead and the mental flexibility that makes it possible to juggle priorities effectively are both likely important in maintaining an exercise routine. Individuals who are cognitively strained, or depleted, may have difficulty engaging in healthy behaviors.[8]

Self-regulation develops during childhood and can set the stage for adult self-regulation capacity.[9,10] In adults, self-regulation deficits are linked to poor chronic health conditions, including obesity, which often require long-term behavior and lifestyle changes in order to manage.[11] Identifying how self-regulation processes that emerge early in life relate to health behaviors is therefore a critical first step toward interventions that address mechanisms of behavior change. Furthermore, improving self-regulation processes early in the lifespan may provide a novel, prevention-oriented approach to health promotion.

EXECUTIVE FUNCTIONING IN CHILDREN

Executive functioning (EF) is a central aspect of self-regulation. EF refers to a set of interrelated neurocognitive functions that concern attentional, mental flexibility, and self-control capacities. Such skills emerge rapidly during the early childhood years and continue to develop throughout later childhood and into adolescence.[12] EF skills generally include attention shifting, working memory, and inhibition of prepotent responses, or inhibitory control (**Fig. 1**).[13] These skills function to direct and control cognitive and, to some extent behavioral processes to focus on a task at hand as well as to plan for the future.

EF has both cool and hot components that are activated under conditions that vary in motivational salience.[14] That is, cool features of EF reflect the child's capacity to control

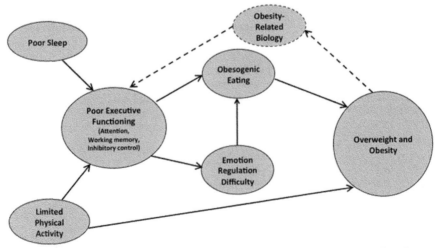

Fig. 1. Potential pathways of association between poor EF and obesity in childhood.

attention and make choices in a situation that does not involve emotional challenge or high-stakes decision making, whereas hot EF skills are important when the child needs to make decisions that are motivationally salient. Cool components of EF thus include working memory and attentional capacity, whereas inhibitory control is considered a hotter EF skill. Cooler EF skills have been associated with the lateral prefrontal cortex, which shapes complex cognitive skills such as planning and attentional flexibility,[15] whereas hotter EF skills have been associated with the orbitofrontal cortex, which is hypothesized to be involved in more affectively salient decision making.[16,17] However, the mapping of EF skills to specific brain structures is still emerging, and the developmental trajectories of cool and hot EF skills are still not fully understood.[18,19]

EF skills have been found to underlie functioning in many domains, including academic achievement (particularly cool EF[20]) and emotion regulation (particularly hot EF[21]) as of early childhood. Both cool and hot components of EF may also have implications for health behaviors, but EF skills have rarely been examined with regard to health-related behaviors in children.

DETERMINANTS OF EXECUTIVE FUNCTIONING IN CHILDREN

Understanding the determinants of EF is important in order to identify opportunities for intervention to enhance EF. The preschool to early school years are a critical period for the development of EF.[12,20] Deficits in EF may arise as a result of toxic stress exposure during early life, which can occur in the context of poverty and is known to have long-lasting effects on brain development and organization.[22] Research has identified both genetic factors[23–25] and early behavioral precursors of EF, including infant and toddler attention skills,[26] emotional reactivity,[27] and sleep.[28] Social-contextual features have been consistently associated with EF capacities, and the importance of parenting has recently been highlighted.[29] Children who are born into poverty,[30,31] experience intrusive parenting,[30,32] or have parents with low EF themselves[33] display reduced EF skills even as early as the preschool years. In contrast, positive caregiving and secure attachment are associated with better early EF skills[32,34] and preschool curricula that provide highly scaffolded, play-based, and predictable social environments can have beneficial effects on EF.[35] As with other developmental phenomena, EF skills are most likely a result of the interplay between genetic and other biological factors and the child's caregiving environment.[27,33,36]

DEVELOPMENT OF EXECUTIVE FUNCTIONING

Taking a developmental perspective is essential in order to understand how EF could shape health behavior. Early childhood is a period of rapid brain growth with constant remodeling of neural architecture and synaptic pruning;[37,38] EF skills thus develop rapidly during this time and there is evidence of malleability.[35,39] EF skills continue to develop across the first 2 decades of life, generally in conjunction with brain maturation.[18] Importantly, not only brain structures but also neural organization and functional connectivity among brain regions change and develop over this time.[37,38] Certain cooler EF skills, such as working memory, may develop earlier than hot EF skills, such as behavioral inhibition, which continue to develop into preadolescence and beyond.[14,18]

Importantly when considering implications for health behavior, demands on EF also change across development as a function of social context.[16] For example, the temptation for adolescents to engage in high-risk activities can increase when with friends, even if the adolescent is cognitively aware of potential negative consequences.[40] Therefore, although adolescents generally possess more developed EF skills than younger children, they are also required to negotiate more complex contexts that test such skills to a greater degree; the failure of EF skills in such settings may therefore be particularly costly to an adolescent's health.[41,42]

POOR EXECUTIVE FUNCTION IS ASSOCIATED WITH CHILDHOOD OBESITY

Obesity and overweight during childhood and adolescence are associated with a wide range of cognitive skill deficits; over the past decade there has been a dramatic increase in the number of articles reporting on the association.[43-51] However, given that few studies have used overlapping measures or assessed the same aspects of EF in similar populations, the precise nature of association between different EF components and weight remains unclear. Among young children (<6 years of age), deficits in hot behavioral inhibition skills have been consistently associated with higher body mass index (BMI) and overweight as assessed using behavioral delay of gratification tasks[52,53] as well as cognitively focused EF tasks.[43,54] Less is known about cool EF skills in relation to weight in children younger than school age. Among older children and adolescents, reduced EF skills in the areas of inhibitory control, attention, and working memory, as well as differences in brain activation in cortical regions associated with reward, have been found in association with overweight and obesity.[46,49,50,55,56] Using longitudinal designs to study associations between EF components and weight across different developmental periods can help identify which aspects of EF are uniquely associated with weight (or other adiposity indicators) and when such associations emerge.

POSSIBLE PATHWAYS OF ASSOCIATION IN CHILDREN

Beyond simply identifying associations between weight and EF, it is important to understand the complex pathways through which EF deficits and obesity become established during childhood in order to recommend intervention approaches. **Fig. 1** presents an overview of EF-obesity pathways that are supported by research evidence to date (note that neither all possible pathways nor all bidirectional arrows are represented). In children, poor EF has been associated with obesity-promoting behaviors, including obesogenic eating, lack of physical activity, emotion regulation difficulties, and poor sleep, although in some cases such behaviors may be driving poor EF performance and/or the associations may be bidirectional (eg, sleep,[57] physical activity,[58] emotion regulation[6]).

Deficits in hot EF skills such as behavioral inhibition have been associated with poorer emotion regulation[21] as well as obesogenic eating behaviors such as emotional overeating,[59] reduced self-regulation of eating,[60] and intake of high-calorie snack foods[61] in preschool and school-aged children, although findings are not consistent, particularly in younger children.[62] Difficulty delaying immediate gratification in favor of long-term goals may be responsible for self-regulation failures in the context of emotional distress or in the presence of tempting foods, which may increase the level of self-regulatory effort involved to delay gratification and therefore the likelihood that a child's capacity to self-regulate will be depleted rapidly.[8] In particular, individuals who are higher in food reward sensitivity or who eat to calm themselves when upset may be highly susceptible to such failures and thereby more prone to obesity.[63,64] However, this possibility has rarely been considered in children; thus, research examining the inhibitory control aspect of EF with regard to food reward and emotion regulation capacity in young children is needed in order to clarify these processes.

Compared with immediate delay of gratification, a hot EF skill, cooler EF capacities such as working memory and planning may operate through a longer-term pathway wherein limited capacities to plan ahead to eat healthfully or exercise, or a lack of focus on future goals, could increase obesity over time. Evidence for this pathway in children is limited, particularly in young children. One study of school-aged children found that cool, but not hot, EF was associated with parent-reported obesogenic eating behavior,[65,66] and another study found that children who reported more sedentary behavior and high snack food intake showed EF deficits in the areas of working memory and organization, whereas lower-risk children did not show such patterns.[67] Findings based on adolescent samples have shown that poor planning ability was associated with increased binge eating in overweight children,[68] and that binge eating mediated longitudinal EF-BMI associations in girls.[69] The implications of cooler versus hotter EF skills for obesity risk may thus change with development. Because adolescents are known to follow peer influences with regard to eating and health behaviors,[70] deficits in either cool EF skills such as planning or hot EF skills driving affectively loaded decision making could increase risk as a function of the peer group.

Regarding other behavioral risk factors for obesity, both cool and hot EF skills have been associated with greater physical activity,[71,72] but most studies in this area focus on how physical activity may improve EF as a pathway for intervention[58,73] rather than on the role of EF in promoting physical activity. Thus, future work that distinguishes the potentially unique roles of cool and hot EF skills in relation to different obesity-promoting behaviors over the short and long term may allow clinicians to tailor developmentally sensitive interventions to reduce obesity risk based on EF as well as obesity risk behavior profiles.

MECHANISMS OF EXECUTIVE FUNCTIONING–PEDIATRIC OBESITY ASSOCIATION ARE POORLY UNDERSTOOD

Although EF-obesity associations are increasingly recognized, the underlying mechanisms are not yet well delineated and the causal direction of association is debated.[44,74,75] Poor EF may contribute to obesity risk by reducing self-regulation capacity, but the association could be bidirectional.[44,55,74] Experimental studies in adults have shown that EF skills, particularly working memory, can improve after dietary changes[76] and surgically induced weight loss.[77] It is difficult to extrapolate from these studies directly to the pediatric context, because most such work has been conducted in older adults who have been overweight for years or in animal models that can identify mechanisms but only approximate human development. However, obesity-related biology has been proposed to contribute to reduced cognitive function through inflammatory and appetite-regulating hormone–mediated pathways (indicated by the dashed line in **Fig. 1**).[74] Mechanistic and experimental work is needed in children in order to determine the direction of association and inform intervention strategies. For example, intervening to enhance EF may change behavioral pathways leading from poor EF to obesity, whereas reducing adiposity-related factors that impair cognitive skills (eg, through physical activity or surgical interventions) could interrupt the harmful effects of obesity on EF.

INTERVENTION IMPLICATIONS

The literature reviewed earlier suggests multiple implications and directions for intervention. Researchers have attempted to improve EF in children using a variety of approaches (**Fig. 2**). Group-based[78] and classroom-based curriculum interventions[35] that take a comprehensive approach to developing and supporting broad aspects of self-regulation have been shown to be effective in enhancing EF in young children. Given the known associations between parenting and EF,[29] incorporating a focus on parenting in future work in this area may also be helpful. Few obesity prevention

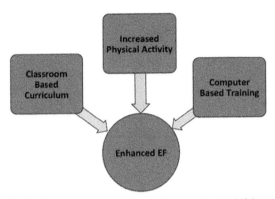

Fig. 2. Effective behavioral strategies to enhance EF capacity in children.

studies have focused on EF skills. However, some work using this type of approach found that improving EF-related capacities in school settings in combination with nutrition-focused content showed positive effects on eating behavior[79] and motor skill development,[80] although not weight.

Physical activity interventions have also shown promise in enhancing EF skills among school-aged overweight children,[81,82] and cognitively engaging exercise has been suggested to be uniquely beneficial.[73] Increasing physical activity may have dual benefit by not only enhancing EF but also directly reducing obesity risk through promoting physical activity. Thus, further examination and testing of such interventions is warranted.

More targeted approaches, such as computer-based EF training programs, that promote skills such as working memory and cognitive flexibility have also been shown to improve EF among school-aged children (7–10 years)[83] and preschoolers,[84–86] as well as in clinical populations of children with attention-deficit/hyperactivity disorder.[39,87,88] There is debate regarding the level of transfer across tasks (eg, whether training cool EF skills also changes hot EF skills),[89,90] but in general such approaches can be implemented easily and thus may be a useful new direction to try in obesity prevention interventions. In addition, given the increasing evidence for EF-eating behavior associations, EF has been proposed as a method to combat obesity specifically through reducing impulsive overeating behavior pathways.[91,92] Studies in adults and older children that have enhanced EF skills in the context of obesity treatment[93] or trained inhibitory responses specifically in relation to tempting foods[92,94,95] have shown promise in this area. Therefore, computer-mediated EF training interventions that also take food reward sensitivity into account, particularly if they are delivered in a context that could address risk factors in the children's broader social context, could also be a helpful new tool for preventing childhood obesity.

SUMMARY/DISCUSSION

Overall, incorporating a focus on self-regulation processes, particularly EF skills, is an promising potential new direction for interventions that seek to prevent obesity in children. Important considerations for future work include identifying directional pathways of association between EF and obesity-promoting behaviors, and tailoring intervention approaches to address developmental as well as individual child needs. For example, children who are more sensitive to food reward may need an intervention that addresses the ability to inhibit behavioral responses and delay gratification in a tempting food context, whereas other children may benefit from general EF training to enhance long-range planning skills. In addition, intervention efforts that focus on multiple aspects of each child's context and include not only a focus on the individual child but also consider parenting and school settings are likely to have the strongest impact.

REFERENCES

1. Ogden CL, Carroll MD, Kit BK, et al. Prevalence of childhood and adult obesity in the United States, 2011-2012. JAMA 2014;311(8):806–14.
2. Nader P, O'Brien M, Houts R, et al. Identifying risk for obesity in early childhood. Pediatrics 2006;118:e594–601.
3. Summerbell C, Waters E, Edmunds L, et al. Interventions for preventing obesity in children. Cochrane Database Syst Rev 2009;(3):CD001871.
4. Onken LS. Cognitive training: targeting cognitive processes in the development of behavioral interventions. Clin Psychol Sci 2015;3(1):39–44.
5. Mischel W, Shoda Y, Rodriguez ML. Delay of gratification in children. Science 1989;244(4907):933–8.
6. Blair C, Ursache A. A bidirectional model of executive functions and self-regulation. Handbook of self-regulation: research, theory, and applications. 2nd edition. New York: Guilford Press; 2011. p. 300–20.
7. Baumeister RF, Heatherton TF. Self-regulation failure: an overview. Psychol Inq 1996;7(1):1–15.
8. Hagger MS, Panetta G, Leung CM, et al. Chronic inhibition, self-control and eating behavior: test of a 'resource depletion' model. PLoS One 2013;8(10): e76888.
9. Posner MI, Rothbart MK. Developing mechanisms of self-regulation. Dev Psychopathol 2000;12(03):427–41.
10. Kochanska G, Coy KC, Murray KT. The development of self-regulation in the first four years of life. Child Dev 2001;72(4):1091–111.
11. Heatherton TF, Wagner DD. Cognitive neuroscience of self-regulation failure. Trends Cogn Sci 2011;15(3):132–9.
12. Davidson MC, Amso D, Anderson LC, et al. Development of cognitive control and executive functions from 4 to 13 years: evidence from manipulations of memory, inhibition, and task switching. Neuropsychologia 2006;44(11):2037–78.
13. Miyake A, Friedman NP, Emerson MJ, et al. The unity and diversity of executive functions and their contributions to complex "Frontal Lobe" tasks: a latent variable analysis. Cognit Psychol 2000;41(1):49–100.
14. Zelazo PD, Carlson SM. Hot and cool executive function in childhood and adolescence: development and plasticity. Child Dev Perspect 2012;6(4):354–60.
15. Miller EK, Cohen JD. An integrative theory of prefrontal cortex function. Annu Rev Neurosci 2001;24(1):167–202.
16. Nelson EE, Guyer AE. The development of the ventral prefrontal cortex and social flexibility. Dev Cogn Neurosci 2011;1(3):233–45.
17. Kringelbach ML. The human orbitofrontal cortex: linking reward to hedonic experience. Nat Rev Neurosci 2005;6(9):691–702.
18. Prencipe A, Kesek A, Cohen J, et al. Development of hot and cool executive function during the transition to adolescence. J Exp Child Psychol 2011;108(3): 621–37.
19. Wiebe SA, Sheffield T, Nelson JM, et al. The structure of executive function in 3-year-olds. J Exp Child Psychol 2011;108(3):436–52.

20. Best JR, Miller PH, Jones LL. Executive functions after age 5: changes and correlates. Dev Rev 2009;29(3):180–200.
21. Blair C. Stress and the development of self-regulation in context. Child Dev Perspect 2010;4(3):181–8.
22. Luby JL. Poverty's most insidious damage: the developing brain. JAMA Pediatr 2015;169(9):810–1.
23. Diamond A, Briand L, Fossella J, et al. Genetic and neurochemical modulation of prefrontal cognitive functions in children. Am J Psychiatry 2004;161(1):125–32.
24. Friedman NP, Miyake A, Young SE, et al. Individual differences in executive functions are almost entirely genetic in origin. J Exp Psychol Gen 2008;137(2):201–25.
25. Logue SF, Gould TJ. The neural and genetic basis of executive function: attention, cognitive flexibility, and response inhibition. Pharmacol Biochem Behav 2014; 123:45–54.
26. Rose SA, Feldman JF, Jankowski JJ. Implications of infant cognition for executive functions at age 11. Psychol Sci 2012;23(11):1345–55.
27. Ursache A, Blair C, Stifter C, et al. Emotional reactivity and regulation in infancy interact to predict executive functioning in early childhood. Dev Psychol 2013; 49(1):127–37.
28. Bernier A, Matte-Gagné C, Bouvette-Turcot A-A. Examining the interface of children's sleep, executive functioning, and caregiving relationships: a plea against silos in the study of biology, cognition, and relationships. Curr Dir Psychol Sci 2014;23(4):284–9.
29. Fay-Stammbach T, Hawes DJ, Meredith P. Parenting influences on executive function in early childhood: a review. Child Dev Perspect 2014;8(4):258–64.
30. Rhoades BL, Greenberg MT, Lanza ST, et al. Demographic and familial predictors of early executive function development: contribution of a person-centered perspective. J Exp Child Psychol 2011;108(3):638–62.
31. Noble KG, McCandliss BD, Farah MJ. Socioeconomic gradients predict individual differences in neurocognitive abilities. Dev Sci 2007;10(4):464–80.
32. Hughes CH, Ensor RA. How do families help or hinder the emergence of early executive function? New Dir Child Adolesc Dev 2009;2009(123):35–50.
33. Deater-Deckard K. Family matters: intergenerational and interpersonal processes of executive function and attentive behavior. Curr Dir Psychol Sci 2014;23(3):230–6.
34. Bernier A, Carlson SM, Deschênes M, et al. Social factors in the development of early executive functioning: a closer look at the caregiving environment. Dev Sci 2012;15(1):12–24.
35. Diamond A, Barnett WS, Thomas J, et al. Preschool program improves cognitive control. Science 2007;318(5855):1387–8.
36. Rochette É, Bernier A. Parenting and preschoolers' executive functioning: a case of differential susceptibility? Int J Behav Dev 2014;40(2):151–61.
37. Casey BJ, Tottenham N, Liston C, et al. Imaging the developing brain: what have we learned about cognitive development? Trends Cogn Sci 2005;9(3):104–10.
38. Gogtay N, Giedd JN, Lusk L, et al. Dynamic mapping of human cortical development during childhood through early adulthood. Proc Natl Acad Sci U S A 2004; 101(21):8174–9.
39. Kray J, Karbach J, Haenig S, et al. Can task-switching training enhance executive control functioning in children with attention deficit/-hyperactivity disorder? Front Hum Neurosci 2011;5:180.
40. Smith AR, Chein J, Steinberg L. Peers increase adolescent risk taking even when the probabilities of negative outcomes are known. Dev Psychol 2014;50(5):1564–8.

41. Blakemore SJ, Choudhury S. Development of the adolescent brain: implications for executive function and social cognition. J Child Psychol Psychiatry 2006; 47(3–4):296–312.

42. Blakemore SJ, Mills KL. Is adolescence a sensitive period for sociocultural processing? Annu Rev Psychol 2014;65:187–207.

43. Guxens M, Mendez MA, Julvez J, et al. Cognitive function and overweight in preschool children. Am J Epidemiol 2009;170(4):438–46.

44. Smith E, Hay P, Campbell L, et al. A review of the association between obesity and cognitive function across the lifespan: Implications for novel approaches to prevention and treatment. Obes Rev 2011;12(9):740–55.

45. Liang J, Matheson BE, Kaye WH, et al. Neurocognitive correlates of obesity and obesity-related behaviors in children and adolescents. Int J Obes 2013;5(10):142.

46. Li Y, Dai Q, Jackson JC, et al. Overweight is associated with decreased cognitive functioning among school-age children and adolescents. Obesity 2008;16(8): 1809–15.

47. Kamijo K, Pontifex MB, Khan NA, et al. The negative association of childhood obesity to cognitive control of action monitoring. Cereb Cortex 2014;24(3): 654–62.

48. Cserjési R, Molnár D, Luminet O, et al. Is there any relationship between obesity and mental flexibility in children? Appetite 2007;49(3):675–8.

49. Lokken KL, Boeka AG, Austin HM, et al. Evidence of executive dysfunction in extremely obese adolescents: a pilot study. Surg Obes Relat Dis 2009;5(5): 547–52.

50. Barkin SL. The relationship between executive function and obesity in children and adolescents: a systematic literature review. J Obes 2013;2013:820956.

51. Khan N, Raine L, Drollette E, et al. Differences in cognitive flexibility between healthy weight and obese children: an ERP study (629.6). FASEB J 2014;28(1 Supplement).

52. Seeyave DM, Coleman S, Appugliese D, et al. Ability to delay gratification at age 4 years and risk of overweight at age 11 years. Arch Pediatr Adolesc Med 2009; 163(4):303–8.

53. Francis LA, Susman EJ. Self-regulation and rapid weight gain in children from age 3 to 12 years. Arch Pediatr Adolesc Med 2009;163(4):297–302.

54. Nederkoorn C, Braet C, Van Eijs Y, et al. Why obese children cannot resist food: the role of impulsivity. Eat Behav 2006;7(4):315–22.

55. Liang J, Matheson BE, Kaye WH, et al. Neurocognitive correlates of obesity and obesity-related behaviors in children and adolescents. Int J Obes 2014;38(4): 494–506.

56. Maayan L, Hoogendoorn C, Sweat V, et al. Disinhibited eating in obese adolescents is associated with orbitofrontal volume reductions and executive dysfunction. Obesity 2011;19(7):1382–7.

57. Sadeh A, Gruber R, Raviv A. The effects of sleep restriction and extension on school-age children: what a difference an hour makes. Child Dev 2003;74(2): 444–55.

58. Hillman CH, Castelli DM, Buck SM. Aerobic fitness and neurocognitive function in healthy preadolescent children. Med Sci Sports Exerc 2005;37(11):1967.

59. Pieper JR, Laugero KD. Preschool children with lower executive function may be more vulnerable to emotional-based eating in the absence of hunger. Appetite 2013;62:103–9.

60. Tan CC, Holub SC. Children's self-regulation in eating: associations with inhibitory control and parents' feeding behavior. J Pediatr Psychol 2011;36(3):340–5.

61. Riggs NR, Spruijt-Metz D, Sakuma K-L, et al. Executive cognitive function and food intake in children. J Nutr Educ Behav 2010;42(6):398–403.
62. Hughes SO, Power TG, O'Connor TM, et al. Executive functioning, emotion regulation, eating self-regulation, and weight status in low-income preschool children: how do they relate? Appetite 2015;89:1–9.
63. van den Berg L, Pieterse K, Malik JA, et al. Association between impulsivity, reward responsiveness and body mass index in children. Int J Obes (Lond) 2011;35(10):1301–7.
64. Nederkoorn C, Houben K, Hofmann W, et al. Control yourself or just eat what you like? weight gain over a year is predicted by an interactive effect of response inhibition and implicit preference for snack foods. Health Psychol 2010;29(4): 389–93.
65. Groppe K, Elsner B. Executive function and food approach behavior in middle childhood. Front Psychol 2014;5:447.
66. Groppe K, Elsner B. The influence of hot and cool executive function on the development of eating styles related to overweight in children. Appetite 2015; 87(0):127–36.
67. Riggs N, Huh J, Chou C-P, et al. Executive function and latent classes of childhood obesity risk. J Behav Med 2012;35(6):642–50.
68. Manasse SM, Juarascio AS, Forman EM, et al. Executive functioning in overweight individuals with and without loss-of-control eating. Eur Eat Disord Rev 2014;22(5):373–7.
69. Goldschmidt AB, Hipwell AE, Stepp SD, et al. Weight gain, executive functioning, and eating behaviors among girls. Pediatrics 2015;136(4):e856–63.
70. Story M, Neumark-Sztainer D, French S. Individual and environmental influences on adolescent eating behaviors. J Am Diet Assoc 2002;102(3 Supplement): S40–51.
71. Riggs N, Chou C-P, Spruijt-Metz D, et al. Executive cognitive function as a correlate and predictor of child food intake and physical activity. Child Neuropsychol 2010;16(3):279–92.
72. Riggs NR, Spruijt-Metz D, Chou C-P, et al. Relationships between executive cognitive function and lifetime substance use and obesity-related behaviors in fourth grade youth. Child Neuropsychol 2012;18(1):1–11.
73. Best JR. Effects of physical activity on children's executive function: contributions of experimental research on aerobic exercise. Dev Rev 2010;30(4):331–51.
74. Miller AL, Lee HJ, Lumeng JC. Obesity-associated biomarkers and executive function in children. Pediatr Res 2014;77(1–2):143–7.
75. Tandon P, Thompson S, Moran L, et al. Body mass index mediates the effects of low income on preschool children's executive control, with implications for behavior and academics. Child Obes 2015;11(5):569–76.
76. Edwards LM, Murray AJ, Holloway CJ, et al. Short-term consumption of a high-fat diet impairs whole-body efficiency and cognitive function in sedentary men. FASEB J 2011;25(3):1088–96.
77. Gunstad J, Strain G, Devlin MJ, et al. Improved memory function 12 weeks after bariatric surgery. Surg Obes Relat Dis 2011;7(4):465–72.
78. Traverso L, Viterbori P, Usai MC. Improving executive function in childhood: evaluation of a training intervention for 5-year-old children. Front Psychol 2015;6:525.
79. Riggs NR, Sakuma K-LK, Pentz MA. Preventing risk for obesity by promoting self-regulation and decision-making skills: pilot results from the PATHWAYS to health program (PATHWAYS). Eval Rev 2007;31(3):287–310.

80. Winter SM, Sass DA. Healthy & ready to learn: examining the efficacy of an early approach to obesity prevention and school readiness. J Res Child Educ 2011; 25(3):304–25.
81. Davis CL, Tomporowski PD, McDowell JE, et al. Exercise improves executive function and achievement and alters brain activation in overweight children: a randomized, controlled trial. Health Psychol 2011;30(1):91–8.
82. Krafft CE, Schwarz NF, Chi L, et al. An 8-month randomized controlled exercise trial alters brain activation during cognitive tasks in overweight children. Obesity 2014;22(1):232–42.
83. Wass SV. Applying cognitive training to target executive functions during early development. Child Neuropsychol 2014;21(2):150–66.
84. Rueda MR, Checa P, Combita LM. Enhanced efficiency of the executive attention network after training in preschool children: immediate changes and effects after two months. Dev Cogn Neurosci 2012;2:S192–204.
85. Espinet SD, Anderson JE, Zelazo PD. Reflection training improves executive function in preschool-age children: Behavioral and neural effects. Dev Cogn Neurosci 2013;4:3–15.
86. Dowsett SM, Livesey DJ. The development of inhibitory control in preschool children: effects of "executive skills" training. Dev Psychobiol 2000;36(2):161–74.
87. Chacko A, Bedard AC, Marks DJ, et al. A randomized clinical trial of Cogmed Working Memory Training in school-age children with ADHD: a replication in a diverse sample using a control condition. J Child Psychol Psychiatry 2014; 55(3):247–55.
88. Holmes J, Gathercole SE, Dunning DL. Adaptive training leads to sustained enhancement of poor working memory in children. Dev Sci 2009;12(4):F9–15.
89. Baniqued PL, Kranz MB, Voss MW, et al. Cognitive training with casual video games: points to consider. Front Psychol 2014;4:1010.
90. Thorell LB, Lindqvist S, Bergman Nutley S, et al. Training and transfer effects of executive functions in preschool children. Dev Sci 2009;12(1):106–13.
91. Juarascio AS, Manasse SM, Espel HM, et al. Could training executive function improve treatment outcomes for eating disorders? Appetite 2015;90:187–93.
92. Allom V, Mullan B. Two inhibitory control training interventions designed to improve eating behaviour and determine mechanisms of change. Appetite 2015;89:282–90.
93. Verbeken S, Braet C, Goossens L, et al. Executive function training with game elements for obese children: a novel treatment to enhance self-regulatory abilities for weight-control. Behav Res Ther 2013;51(6):290–9.
94. Houben K, Jansen A. Chocolate equals stop. Chocolate-specific inhibition training reduces chocolate intake and go associations with chocolate. Appetite 2015;87: 318–23.
95. Yokum S, Stice E. Cognitive regulation of food craving: effects of three cognitive reappraisal strategies on neural response to palatable foods. Int J Obes 2013; 37(12):1565–70.

Physical Activity Interventions for Neurocognitive and Academic Performance in Overweight and Obese Youth: A Systematic Review

Eduardo E. Bustamante, PhD[a], Celestine F. Williams, MS[b],
Catherine L. Davis, PhD, FTOS[c],*

KEYWORDS

- Physical activity • Exercise • Childhood obesity • Brain • Cognition
- Executive function • Academic performance • Health disparities

KEY POINTS

- One-third of US children are overweight or obese and typically inactive, with poorer cognition and achievement than their peers; minorities have disparities on these factors.
- Physically active academic lessons seem to benefit cognition and academic performance in overweight and obese children more than normal-weight children.
- A few randomized trials have demonstrated efficacy of regular physical activity for improving cognitive and neurologic outcomes in overweight and obese children, including minorities.
- Improved executive function and increased physical activity might be mutually enhancing; more translational research is needed to harness this potential.
- These findings warrant promotion of physical activity for children, with emphasis on participation of overweight and obese children and minorities. T2 translation research is needed.

Disclosure Statement: The authors report no funding and no conflicts of interest.
Registration: PROSPERO: International prospective register of systematic reviews. 2016: CRD42016032340.
[a] Department of Kinesiology & Nutrition, College of Applied Health Sciences, University of Illinois at Chicago, 1919 West Taylor Street, Room 626, MC 517, Chicago, IL 60516, USA;
[b] Georgia Prevention Institute, Augusta University, 1125 15th Street, HS-1755, Augusta, GA 30912, USA; [c] Department of Pediatrics, Georgia Prevention Institute, Medical College of Georgia, Augusta University, 1125 15th Street, HS-1711, Augusta, GA 30912, USA
* Corresponding author.
E-mail address: cadavis@augusta.edu

INTRODUCTION

In the United States, 18% of children and adolescents are obese[1] with increasing rates of severe obesity.[2] Fully one-third of students are already overweight or obese in elementary school,[1] and these children are at high risk for chronic diseases,[3] evidence low rates of physical activity[3,4] and physical fitness,[5] and perhaps most concerning, decrements in brain structure,[6,7] cognitive function,[8–13] and academic performance[14–17] relative to normal-weight peers. Research on the impact of physical activity, both transient effects of single bouts and durable effects from prolonged training, in overweight and obese children are of special interest to children, parents, clinicians, educators, and policy makers because of their potential to improve health and academics. Increasing emphasis on standardized testing has reduced physical activity offerings at school, where children spend most of their waking time.[18] Unfortunately, minority youth from underserved communities evidence substantially higher rates of overweight, obesity, and chronic disease, with fewer opportunities for physical activity, and perform worse on measures of classroom behavior, cognitive function, and academic performance than their peers.[19–22]

This article focuses on T1 translation (efficacy) of physical activity interventions for neurologic, cognitive, and academic outcomes in overweight and obese children, with attention to minority representation. There is other T1 literature on physical activity in older adults,[23,24] typically developing children,[25–27] and children with attention-deficit/hyperactivity disorder.[28–30] Research in overweight and obese youth is of interest for two main reasons: overweight and obese youth are a population in which researchers are likely to observe the impact of exercise training on children's cognition because of lower levels of the dependent variable (ie, aspects of cognitive function are impaired in children that are overweight or obese relative to normal weight peers)[31] and low exposure to the independent variable (ie, physical activity and fitness levels are lower in overweight or obese children relative to children without these conditions); and evidence specific to overweight and obese youth is important to meet the growing needs presented by this epidemic.

The rationale for this area of research derives from basic research demonstrating benefits of physical activity on brain function and cognitive performance in rats[32]; and observational studies establishing associations between physical activity, physical fitness, and weight status with brain function, cognitive function, and academic performance.[33–35] Executive function, including core elements of inhibition, working memory, and cognitive flexibility, which together enable complex decision making, self-monitoring, and planning functions,[36] is poorer in obese children and adolescents,[31] and is more responsive to physical activity than other cognitive abilities, such as memory.[24,37,38]

METHODS

A systematic review of the literature was conducted.[39] See **Box 1** for details.

RESULTS
Acute Bout Studies

To date, there have been three studies investigating the impact of acute (single) bouts of physical activity on cognition and academic performance in overweight and obese school-age children.[40–42] All three used within-subjects designs counterbalancing bouts of physical activity with bouts of sedentary time. Methodologic rigor was low to moderate (no randomization, or analyses ignored cluster randomization; per

> **Box 1**
> **Selection criteria**
>
> - PubMed, Journals@OVID, and Web of Science were searched electronically
> - Search key words: *children* with either *exercise* or *physical activity*, with either *overweight, obese, weight status, body mass index*, and either *cognition, brain function, neurologic function, cognitive function, executive function*, or *academics*
> - Inclusion criteria
>   - Paper written in English
>   - Published in a peer-reviewed journal before December 2015
>   - Participants were exclusively overweight or obese children, or outcomes were reported on overweight or obese children separately
>   - Intervention was either one acute bout, or at least several weeks of regular exercise, physical activity, or sport
>   - Neurologic, cognitive, or academic outcomes were reported
>   - Empirical study designs
>   - Acute bout
>   - Quasi-experimental
>   - Randomized controlled trials
> - Using these search terms and inclusion criteria, 13,740 records were identified
> - After eligibility screening, 17 records from 12 studies were included in the systematic review **(Fig. 1)**
> - A summary of study results is found in **Table 1**

protocol analyses). Among these, two investigated effects of 10- to 15-minute physically active versus sedentary academic lessons on normal-weight and overweight or obese children,[40,42] whereas the third investigated the impacts of a 23-minute bout of moderate-intensity treadmill walking among overweight and obese children.[41] Race or ethnicity was reported in two of these studies, one with a majority African American sample[41] and the other a majority white sample.[40] Studies of active academic lessons yielded group × time × weight status findings on reaction time for an inhibition task[42] and time-on-task in classroom observations,[40] such that overweight and obese children generated a greater benefit from the physically active lessons relative to the sedentary lessons when compared with normal-weight children. In contrast, the bout of treadmill walking did not result in any significant differences between groups in cognitive outcomes.[41]

Regular Physical Activity

Quasi-experimental studies

Four quasi-experimental studies of regular physical activity effects on cognition in overweight and obese youth tested 8-week to 1-year interventions combining physical activity with other lifestyle elements.[43–48] These studies had low rigor (no control group for intervention). Delgado-Rico and coworkers[43] showed improvements after a 12-week, weekly lifestyle intervention in Spain on adolescents' impulsive behavior and a Stroop task, and correlated reduced body mass index with improvements in cognitive outcomes. Kinder and colleagues[44] tested 45 weeks of sports therapy and health education on functional MRI (fMRI) activation during exposure to images. Only youth that lost weight (responders) showed changes in activation in response to images of food and sport following the intervention.[44] Vanhelst and colleagues[48] showed improvements on teacher ratings following 1 year of weekly physical activity sessions and quarterly health classes in France. However, very similar results

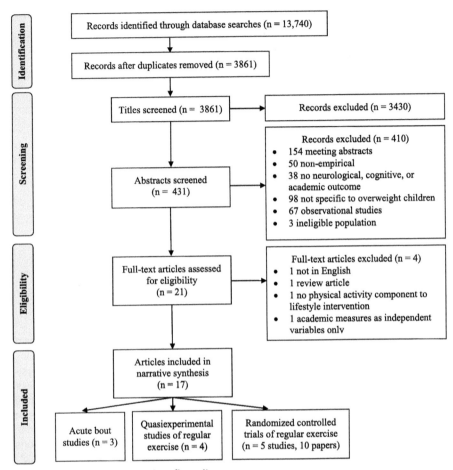

Fig. 1. PRISMA systematic review flow diagram.

appeared in other reports from this study, with inconsistent intervention descriptions (1 or 2 years, monthly or quarterly health classes), which reduces confidence in the results.[45,46] Kulendran and colleagues[47] compared normal-weight control subjects with overweight and obese youth who underwent an 8-week day camp, including daily sport participation. Overweight and obese youth improved on prespecified primary outcomes of inhibition and impulsivity after intervention; no posttest data were collected from control subjects.[47] None of these quasi-experimental studies reported participant race or ethnicity.

Randomized controlled trials

Ten publications from five randomized controlled trials (RCTs) have investigated the impact of regular physical activity on neurologic, cognitive, or academic function in overweight or obese youth, with methodologic rigor ranging from low to high.[38,49–57]

The first trial, nicknamed the "PLAY Project," randomized a community sample of 222 overweight or obese children (majority African American) into three groups: (1) high-dose group (40 minutes of exercise training per day after school), (2) low-dose group (20 minutes of exercise training per day after school), or (3) a no-intervention group for 13 ± 1.6 weeks.[38,50,58] This study is unique because it tested a

Table 1
Physical activity intervention studies with neurologic, cognitive, and academic outcomes in overweight and obese children

Source	Study Design	Participants	Intervention	Time Points	Results[a]	Rigor
Acute bouts of physical activity						
Grieco et al,[40] 2009	Cluster-randomized design (order of active vs sedentary lesson was randomized by classroom)	Nine third-grade classrooms including 97 children; 64% normal weight, 20% overweight, 17% obese; 69% white, 14% Hispanic, 11% African American, 6% Asian	One 10- to 15-min academic lesson, "Texas I-CAN," delivered through moderate to vigorous physical activity vs sedentary lesson, on 2 non-PE days	Baseline, posttest	Academic outcome • Time-on-task at posttest[b]	2

Tomporowski et al,[37,41] 2008	Within-subject counterbalanced order design compared treadmill walking vs educational video	N = 69, 7–11 y old; 100% overweight or obese; 55% African American, 45% white	23-min treadmill walking (4-min warm-up, 15 min at 3 mph and 3% grade, 4-min cool down) vs 23-min video watching, on 2 d with 5.5 ± 1.2 d between visits	Baseline, posttest	Cognitive outcomes
					• **Switch task**
					  ○ **Response time**
					  ○ Accuracy
						2

Vazou and Smiley-Oyen,[42] 2014	Within-subjects design counterbalancing a physically active math lesson with a seated math lesson	N = 35 third to fifth grade students; 31% overweight or obese; race or ethnicity not reported	20-min reading to induce fatigue, followed by "Move for Thought" 10-min bout of aerobic physical activity integrated with math practice vs seated math lesson, on 2 d with 7.8 ± 2 d between visits	Baseline, posttest	Cognitive outcomes
					• Flanker
					  ○ Standard (inhibition)
					    ■ Reaction time[b,c]
					    ■ Accuracy
					  ○ Reverse (inhibition + switching)
					    ■ Reaction time
					    ■ Accuracy
					  ○ Mixed (inhibition + switching + working memory)
					    ■ Reaction time
					    ■ Accuracy
						1

(continued on next page)

Table 1
(continued)

Source	Study Design	Participants	Intervention	Time Points	Results[a]	Rigor
Regular physical activity						
Quasi-experimental						

Vanhelst et al,[45,48] 2012, 2010[46]	Single group (uncontrolled)	N = 37, 7–17 years old, 100% obese, race/ethnicity not reported	2-h physical activity sessions were offered once per week for 12 mo; 1-h health education program was offered every 3 mo	Baseline, posttest	Academic outcomes
					• Teacher interview
					  ○ Changes in class standing
					  ○ Self-esteem[d]
					  ○ Self-evaluation of academic performance[d]
					  ○ Ability to work alone[d]
						1

Kinder et al,[44] 2014	Single group (uncontrolled), compared responders with nonresponders (children who lost weight vs those who did not) post hoc	N = 14 who provided fMRI data, 7–15 y old, 100% overweight or obese, race/ethnicity not reported (three usable fMRI scans from children who gained weight were excluded for matching)	Therapeutic interventions (sports therapy, physical and dietary education) twice per week for 45 wk	Baseline, posttest	Neurologic outcome
					• fMRI BOLD activity during exposure to images of food, sport, pleasure, and neutral stimuli
					Comparisons of responders vs nonresponders revealed greater activation in responders at posttest
					  ○ Putamen, in response to food pictures
					  ○ Motor network, in response to sport pictures
						1

Study	Design	Sample	Intervention	Assessment	Cognitive outcomes	
Delgado-Rico et al,[43] 2012	Single group (uncontrolled)	N = 42, 12–17 y old, 100% overweight or obese, race/ethnicity not reported	12-wk lifestyle intervention (one group session/week) with cognitive behavioral therapy, physical activity prescription (≥1 h of moderate-to-vigorous-intensity aerobic exercise 3–5 d/wk) and monitoring, and dietary prescription and monitoring	Baseline, posttest	Cognitive outcomes • UPPS-P Impulsive Behavior Scale ○ Negative Urgency[d] ○ Lack of premeditation ○ Lack of perseverance ○ Sensation seeking ○ Positive urgency • Letter number sequencing • Stroop Color-Word Task ○ Response inhibition ○ Response inhibition and switching[d] ○ Response switching • Iowa Gambling Task	1
Kulendran et al,[47] 2014	Case-control (overweight or obese youth at baseline vs normal-weight control subjects); single group (overweight only) intervention study	N = 53, 10–17 y old, 100% overweight or obese; N = 50 nonobese adolescent control subjects, race/ethnicity not reported	8-wk multidimensional weight loss day camp, including daily team sport participation	Baseline, posttest	Cognitive outcomes • Inhibition ○ Stop-signal task (reaction time)[d] • Impulsivity ○ Delayed discounting task[d]	1

(continued on next page)

Table 1
(continued)

Source	Study Design	Participants	Intervention	Time Points	Results[a]	Rigor
Randomized controlled trials						

Davis et al,[38] 2007, 2011[50]	Three-arm RCT comparing 0-min, 20-min, and 40-min per day of exercise training	N = 171, 8–11 y old, 100% overweight or obese, 61% African American, 39% white	3-mo, 5 d per week, after-school aerobic exercise training (20 or 40 min) program vs no intervention	Baseline, posttest	Cognitive outcomes
					• Cognitive Assessment System
					  ○ Full Scale
					    ■ **Planning**[c]
					    ■ Attention
					    ■ Simultaneous
					    ■ Successive
					Academic outcomes
					• Woodcock-Johnson Tests of Achievement III
					  ○ Broad Reading
					  ○ Broad Math[c]
					Neurologic outcomes
					• **fMRI BOLD activity (N = 20)**
					  ○ Bilateral prefrontal cortex[c]
					  ○ Bilateral posterior parietal cortex[c]
						3

Staiano et al,[49] 2012	Three-arm RCT comparing cooperative vs competitive exergaming vs no intervention	N = 54, 15–19 y old, most of whom were overweight or obese, 100% African American	10-wk daily exergame (competitive vs cooperative) offered 30 min per day (participation averaged 15.5 min once per week), vs no intervention	Baseline, posttest	Cognitive outcomes • Delis-Kaplan Executive Function System[c]	1

Crova et al,[51] 2014	Two-arm cluster RCT compared curricular PE with enhanced PE	Six classes in two schools included 70 children, 9–10 y old, who provided baseline and posttest data; 37% overweight or obese; race/ethnicity not reported	6 mo, 5 d per week, curricular PE plus 2 h/wk of fundamental motor skill, perceptual–motor, and tennis instruction taught by a specialist, vs one curricular PE class/week taught by a generalist	Baseline, posttest	Cognitive outcomes
					• Random **Number** Generation Task
					  ○ Inhibition[e]
					  ○ Working memory
						1

Study	Design	Sample	Intervention	Timing	Outcomes	

Krafft et al,[53] 2014	2-arm RCT comparing exercise vs sedentary attention control condition	N = 43 children who provided baseline and posttest fMRI data, 8–11 y old, 100% overweight or obese, 91% African American, 9% white	8-mo daily after-school aerobic exercise program, 40 min per day vigorous intensity intermittent physical activity (average heart rate 161 bpm) vs similar but sedentary program	Baseline, posttest	Neurologic outcomes
					• **fMRI BOLD response**
					  ○ **Antisaccade task**[c]
					  ○ Flanker task[c]
					Cognitive outcomes
					• Antisaccade performance
					  ○ Accuracy
					• Flanker performance
					  ○ Congruent
					    ■ Accuracy
					  ○ Incongruent
					    ■ Accuracy
					    ■ Interference effect
						2

Krafft et al,[53] 2014	"	N = 22 children who provided baseline and posttest resting fMRI data, 8–11 y old, 100% overweight or obese, 95% African American, 5% white	"	"	Neurologic outcome
					• **fMRI resting state synchrony**
					  ○ Default mode network[c]
					  ○ Cognitive control network[c]
					  ○ Salience network
					  ○ Motor network[c]
						2

Krafft et al,[54] 2014	"	N = 18 children who provided baseline and posttest diffusion tensor imaging data, 8–11 y old, 100% overweight or obese, 94% African American, 6% white	"	"	Neurologic outcomes
					• **White matter integrity**
					  ○ **Superior longitudinal fasciculus**
					    ■ Fractional anisotropy[e]
					    ■ Radial diffusivity[e]
					Cognitive outcomes
					• Behavioral Rating Inventory of Executive Function (teacher rating)
					• Cognitive Assessment System
						2

Schaeffer et al,[56] 2014	"	"	"	"	Neurologic outcomes
					• White matter integrity
					  ○ Uncinate fasciculus
					    ■ Fractional anisotropy[c]
					    ■ Radial diffusivity[c]
						2

(continued on next page)

Table 1
(continued)

Source	Study Design	Participants	Intervention	Time Points	Results[a]	Rigor

Davis et al,[57] 2015	"	N = 175, 8-11 y old, 100% overweight or obese, 84% African American, 16% white	8-mo daily after-school aerobic exercise program, 40 min per day vigorous intensity intermittent physical activity (average heart rate 161 bpm, at an intensity of seven metabolic equivalents, with 59% attendance) vs similar but sedentary program (64% attendance)	Baseline, posttest, 12 mo	Cognitive outcomes
					• **Cognitive Assessment System**
					  ○ **Planning**
					  ○ Attention
					  ○ Simultaneous
					  ○ Successive
					  ○ Full Scale
					• Tower of London
					• Behavioral Rating Inventory of Executive Function (teacher rating)
					• Woodcock-Johnson Tests of Achievement III
					• Criterion-Referenced Competency Tests
						3

					Cognitive outcomes

Huang et al,[52] 2015	Two-arm RCT comparing multicomponent health intervention with standard intervention	N = 115 fifth grade students, 100% overweight or obese, 66% Danish, 34% non-Danish	6-wk day camp, 7 d per week, ≥3 h physical activity per day, followed by a five-session family education intervention over 46 wk, vs one 2-h physical activity session per week over 6 wk	Baseline, posttest, 12 mo	• Stroop Color Word Test
					  ○ Interference
					• Rey Complex Figure Test
					  ○ Copy[c]
					  ○ Recall
					• Behavioral Rating Inventory of Executive Function (parent rating, only at baseline and 12 mo)
					  ○ Behavior Regulation Index
					    ■ Inhibit
					    ■ Shift
					    ■ Emotional control[f]
					  ○ Metacognition Index
					    ■ Initiate
					    ■ Working memory
					    ■ Plan/organize
					    ■ Organization of materials
					    ■ Monitor[f]
					  ○ Global Executive Composite

Abbreviations: fMRI, functional MRI; PE, physical education; RCT, randomized controlled trial.

Rigor refers to the quality of evidence for efficacy (1 = low, 2 = medium, 3 = high).

[a] Prespecified primary outcomes are bolded. Sample size is specified only if subsample was used for secondary outcome.

[b] *P*<.05 group × time × weight status analysis at posttest.

[c] *P*<.05 group × time analysis at posttest.

[d] *P*<.05 within-group analysis for pretest versus posttest, for quasi-experimental studies only.

[e] *P*<.05 group × time × attendance analysis at posttest.

[f] *P*<.05 group × time analysis at follow-up.

dose-response relationship (ie, 0 minutes vs 20 minutes vs 40 minutes per day of vigorous physical activity) using an experimental design rather than post hoc association. Both exercise training groups were well attended, with high daily average heart rates showing vigorous exertion. The exercise treatments reduced fatness, improved fitness, and reduced diabetes risk.[58] At baseline and posttest, cognition and academic achievement was measured, yielding a sample of 171 children with baseline measures, and excellent retention (96%).[50] Results from the planning scale of the cognitive test[59] demonstrated a linear dose-response pattern such that the higher doses of exercise training resulted in better executive function (the prespecified primary outcome in the ancillary study of cognition) at posttest, with a similar dose-response pattern for math achievement.[50] No other cognitive scales, including attention, responded to the program, supporting the hypothesized selective effect of exercise training on more complex executive functions.[23,24,50] Concomitant group differences in change of fMRI brain activation patterns during an inhibition (antisaccade) task were found in a subsample (20 children in an fMRI pilot study), with greater increases in the prefrontal cortex and greater decreases in the posterior parietal cortex in the exercise groups relative to children randomized to the control condition.[50] This was the most rigorous study of exercise effects on children's cognition to date regardless of weight status, because of sample size, a substantial monitored exercise dose, and adherence to CONSORT standards including intent-to-treat analyses and blinded outcome assessors.

Two small RCTs were conducted in overweight and obese youth. One randomized 54 overweight and obese African American adolescents to play interactive exercise video games (ie, exergames) competitively versus cooperatively, or to receive no intervention for 10 weeks.[49] Play sessions were offered each school day. Game play lasted an average of 15.5 minutes per session, and participants played on average one time per week. Adolescents in the competitive condition outperformed the other groups on an executive function test, and weight loss during the intervention was positively correlated with executive function improvement, lending some dose-response evidence. The study did not conduct intent-to-treat analysis or report details of randomization or retention, thus it has moderate rigor. A cluster RCT investigated the impact of cognitively challenging physical activity on executive function in overweight children.[51] Crova and colleagues[51] aimed to test the hypothesis that the cognitive benefits of physical activity derived from the level of cognitive challenge or engagement involved in the activity. This intriguing hypothesis[37,60,61] was tested by randomizing six primary school classrooms at two schools in Italy (37% overweight or obese, race or ethnicity not reported) to receive one standard physical education (PE) class per week, versus standard PE plus 2 hours of cognitively enhanced PE (ie, motor skill training, tennis skills) per week for 6 months. Group × time analyses were not reported; the study posited differences in group × time × weight status, where overweight children would be more likely to benefit from the enhanced PE than normal-weight peers. Overweight children achieved significantly greater gains in inhibition (but not memory updating) from enhanced PE versus standard PE, whereas normal-weight children did not have a group difference; fitness gains were not found to mediate the cognitive benefits.[51] The study, while presenting an interesting hypothesis and mechanistic approach, suffers from confounds with intervention (teacher skill level, time in intervention) and ignored cluster randomization in analysis, and therefore has low rigor.

In 2014, the Davis group published four reports on brain scans from their second RCT of aerobic training for overweight and obese children's cognition and neurologic function.[53–56] The SMART study randomized 175 predominantly African American children to the after-school training program or a comparable, but sedentary attention control program. Each met every school day, for approximately an academic year (8 months). Krafft and colleagues[55] found significant group × time changes in fMRI BOLD activity, a prespecified primary outcome. Consistent with the PLAY project, alterations were found in prefrontal and posterior parietal cortex activation during cognitive tasks (ie, antisaccade and flanker tasks); performance on the tasks did not differ by group. Improved resting-state fMRI results were detected: default mode, cognitive control, and motor networks showed more spatial refinement over time in the exercise group compared with control subjects, suggesting quicker brain maturation in the exercise group.[53] Krafft and colleagues[54] reported null group × time findings on neurologic and cognitive outcomes in a subsample with white matter integrity (WMI) data; however, post hoc analyses revealed group × time × attendance interactions on a primary outcome, superior longitudinal fasciculus WMI, such that attendance to the exercise program was related to greater gains, whereas attendance to the control program was unrelated. Moreover, when participants were clustered by increased WMI in the superior longitudinal fasciculus and those without (regardless of randomization), the WMI-improved children improved on teacher ratings and tests of executive function, showing correspondence between neurobiologic and behavioral changes.[54] Findings in another tract, the uncinate fasciculus, demonstrated a group × time interaction such that participants in the exercise training program demonstrated greater gains in WMI relative to those in the attention control condition.[56] The results of intent-to-treat analyses on the primary and secondary cognitive and achievement outcomes from the full sample at posttest and 12-month follow-up showed null effects overall, indicating that the nonspecific effects of intervention on children's cognition and achievement may be stronger than exercise training effects per se.[57] More precise measurement of neural outcomes may explain the positive findings on these measures versus the null cognition and achievement outcomes.

The most recent trial randomly allocated 115 overweight or obese predominantly Danish fifth graders to a 6-week day camp, including 3 or more hours per day of physical activity or sport, versus one 2-hour physical activity session per week over the same time period.[52] There was a group × time difference showing a camp benefit on the Rey Complex Figure Test Copy Scale at posttest, with no such differences on the figure recall or the Stroop task; no group × time effects were apparent at 1-year follow-up on these tests.[52] However, group × time differences at 1-year follow-up benefiting the camp participants were seen on the Behavioral Rating Inventory of Executive Function parent rating scale (which was not administered at posttest),[62] for two of eight subscales (Emotional Control and Monitor), but no summary scales. To their credit, the authors acknowledged possible parent bias for this result. Apart from those of Davis and colleagues, this study was the only one to provide a participant flowchart, report attendance to the interventions, and conduct intent-to-treat analyses, therefore the posttest analyses are considered to have high rigor. However, the follow-up results are confounded with the family education intervention in one group, reducing confidence in those findings.

DISCUSSION

During an unwavering child obesity epidemic[1] with low levels of physical activity and excessive sedentary time especially in minority and obese children,[63] information about acute and longer-term physical activity intervention effects on cognition, achievement, and brain health is needed to inform policy and clinical practice.

Acute bouts of exercise last only minutes to hours, and result in neurobiologic, cognitive, and affective benefits that are transient, dissipating as quickly as 15 minutes following the bout.[64] Three studies of acute exercise effects on cognition in overweight or obese school-age children were of low to moderate rigor because of small sample size[42] and per-protocol analyses.[40–42] Where cluster randomization was used, analyses ignored the clustering; however, this is not important because the randomization was used to counterbalance order of conditions.[40] There were also notable strengths. All three used within-subjects designs with randomized or counterbalanced order.[40–42] In a sample that included roughly a quarter minority children, Grieco and colleagues[40] used blinded outcome assessors for a very relevant educational measure, time-on-task. These studies yielded some consistent results. One study in overweight and obese children (majority African American) showed null results from a moderate bout of treadmill walking on cognitive flexibility.[41] The authors suggested that shorter bouts of more intense activity might elicit more benefit.[41] Null effects on cognitive flexibility are consistent with Vazou and Smiley-Oyen.[42] Also, acute bouts may improve inhibition rather than cognitive flexibility through improved alertness, via transient increases in blood flow and circulating catecholamine.[37,65,66] Another consistent finding suggests that overweight and obese children may derive more cognitive benefit from physically active lessons versus sedentary lessons than their normal-weight peers (time-on-task,[40] faster reaction time on only the simplest flanker task[42]). This nascent literature in overweight children complements the broader literature where acute bouts of physical activity were found to improve inhibition in youth.[65]

Quasi-experimental studies provide valuable information on the promise of novel interventions, allow study under conditions when RCTs are not feasible, and provide pilot data to determine whether an RCT is warranted.[67] Each of the four quasi-experimental studies of regular physical activity interventions in overweight and obese children showed some benefit of lifestyle interventions including a physical activity component on neural, cognitive, or academic outcomes,[43,44,47,48] but in each case, the physical activity component was confounded with other elements of the interventions. None of these studies compared intervention effects with changes in a control group, thus benefits attributed to intervention could be caused by other factors (eg, practice, maturation, history, and so forth).[67] These quasi-experimental studies are promising, but of low rigor, providing scant evidence for efficacy of physical activity interventions; these studies did not report race or ethnicity of their samples.

Among the identified RCTs, three followed CONSORT guidelines[68] and therefore provided evidence for efficacy.[38,50,52–56] Two small trials are intriguing but had low rigor.[49,51]

The first Davis and colleagues[38,50] trial was a rigorous study demonstrating dose-response effects of a physical activity program on executive function. Because the parent trial was designed to investigate dose-response effects of aerobic training on diabetes risk in overweight and obese children, including a substantial proportion of African Americans, the cognitive and neurologic outcomes reported were ancillary. The findings of benefits of the exercise programs versus no intervention yielded a refined research question: whether the benefit was caused by physical activity or other nonspecific program features, such as attention from adult staff, social interaction, rules, and behavioral incentives.[50]

The next trial by this group[53–56] built on the first by using a sedentary attention control condition to isolate the impact of the aerobic exercise per se from other program elements. The study implemented a longer intervention (8 months vs 3 months) in a predominantly African American sample, and added cognition, brain function, and structure measurements. Primary outcomes were prespecified (planning, fMRI,

WMI). Although neuroimaging revealed beneficial effects of exercise intervention in those children who provided usable brain scans,[53–56] intent-to-treat results were null on cognitive and achievement outcomes.[57] This indicates that exercise intervention programs may be effective mainly because of the organized activities supervised by adults. Also, neuroimaging may be more responsive than cognitive tests to the effects of exercise intervention.[50,55] Although brain structure and function outcomes used per-protocol analyses[53–56], intent-to-treat analyses later confirmed brain activation and uncinate fasciculus WMI results.[69]

Similar null cognitive results emerged in older adults[70] and children with attention-deficit/hyperactivity disorder[29,71] in recent studies using attention control conditions. These studies diverge from those comparing physical activity programs with no-intervention controls,[25–27,38,50] where results decisively favored physical activity programs. The results of the more stringent comparison presented by a sedentary attention control condition indicate that the attention and behavioral structure of a quality after-school program outweigh physical activity effects on these outcomes.

Huang and colleagues[52] conducted a rigorous trial of a multicomponent lifestyle intervention in a reasonably large sample, showing intent-to-treat group × time benefits on parent ratings of executive function (two of eight subscales) and a visual memory test, but null findings on a well-known executive function test. The study largely followed CONSORT guidelines (eg, details of randomization, allocation concealment), and the intervention provided substantial physical activity. The trial had few weaknesses; however, no primary outcome was specified. The authors acknowledged the parent ratings may be biased. The control condition received minimal attention and therefore was similar to a no-treatment control. Because the day camp used a multicomponent health intervention, one cannot determine how much benefit was caused by physical activity versus other elements. Also, this work does not seem to be relevant to US minority populations.

Two small RCTs of regular physical activity tested novel research questions with lower rigor, appropriate for this early stage of research. Staiano and colleagues[49] tested a novel question, and found an advantage for competitive versus cooperative exergaming versus no intervention on executive function in a small sample of African American adolescents; weight loss was related to cognitive improvements. This study was a pilot rather than an efficacy study, so did not meet CONSORT guidelines.[68] Nonetheless, this study, which focused on an at-risk population of minority adolescents, demonstrated a possible mechanistic link between weight loss and cognitive benefits from a physical activity intervention. Crova and colleagues[51] demonstrated a group × time × weight status interaction on inhibition favoring overweight and obese children in enhanced PE versus standard PE. The cognitively engaging nature of enhanced PE was confounded with the training of the PE specialist and additional 2 hours per week of instruction.[51] This study randomized six classes, but because per-protocol analyses did not use the cluster as the unit of analysis, they seem likely to inflate type 1 error.[72,73] Also, race or ethnicity of the sample was not reported. Nonetheless, the finding that overweight and obese children had greater cognitive benefits than normal-weight children from increased physical activity was consistent with acute bout studies.[40,42] The study also tested, and did not support, mediation of cognitive benefits by improved fitness.[51]

A recent Cochrane review of lifestyle intervention effects on academic outcomes in overweight or obese children and adolescents[74] evaluated two RCTs included in this review[49,50] and four cluster randomized trials that did not meet our inclusion criteria,[12,75–77] excluding several studies included here.[40,41,43,48] Unfortunately, although inclusion of minorities was reported, the meta-analysis failed to standardize effect sizes, rendering study comparisons invalid.[74]

SUMMARY AND FUTURE DIRECTIONS

A few consistent findings across studies of acute bouts and regular exercise emerged from this review. Overweight and obese children may be more cognitively responsive to physical activity interventions than normal-weight children.[40,42,51] This supports the focus of exercise-cognition research on overweight and obese children who stand to benefit more, cognitively and in improving overall health. Acute studies showed that physically active academic lessons benefit inhibition more than cognitive flexibility,[40–42] with partial correspondence among studies of regular physical activity (but see Refs.[50,57]).[47,52]

Public health guidelines for evidence-based practice require at least two quality RCTs to establish efficacy.[78] High-quality RCTs with overweight and obese children have shown benefits of regular physical activity for different executive function[50,52] and neurologic outcomes[50,53–56] in overweight and obese children. However, all the studies showing neurologic benefits were from the same group.[50,53–56] The independent study found executive function benefits only on parent rating subscales.[52] More high-quality trials are needed to establish efficacy of regular exercise for cognitive and brain benefits in overweight or obese children, particularly for minority racial or ethnic groups. A recent meta-analysis found insufficient evidence for efficacy of regular exercise on executive function in children, adolescents, and young adults, without regard to weight status.[65] Indeed, this literature reflects the challenges in conducting intervention research, and highlights the need for greater investment in rigorous clinical trial methodology to strengthen the evidence base in this burgeoning field. Nonetheless, the literature on physical activity effects on cognition and related outcomes in overweight and obese children is as well developed as that of any group other than older adults, and is consistent with results of regular exercise in typically developing children. A recent trial was the first to report a cognitive flexibility benefit of regular exercise versus no intervention in children, many of whom seemed to be overweight or obese, based on their mean body mass index (19 kg/m^2) and age (8.8 years).[25] This study did not meet our inclusion criteria for analyzing children by weight status.

Despite frequently invoked candidate mechanisms, such as fitness and neurotrophins,[34] prespecified mediators have not been empirically confirmed in this literature,[51,79] with the exception of increased WMI linked with executive function improvements.[54] The extent to which physical activity effects on neurocognition is moderated by such factors as sex, race or ethnicity, or other genetic factors remains largely unknown. Although there are a few studies on these factors, there has been little investigation of qualitative aspects of physical activity that may influence cognitive effects, including type (aerobic vs resistance training), intensity, timing (ie, session duration, weekly frequency, and length of participation),[50] mode (eg, swimming vs gymnastics), novelty and cognitive challenge,[36,60,80] setting,[81] social interaction (group vs solitary),[82] behavior management strategies (rules, incentives, consequences),[50,57,83] and mastery experiences.[60]

A promising new area investigates whether the reciprocal effects of executive function, health behavior, and obesity can be harnessed effectively for obesity treatment and prevention. Impaired executive function may promote obesity and decrease physical activity participation.[84,85] Executive function is essential for self-regulation, including health behavior, such as physical activity and sedentary behavior.[85] Better executive function predicts better health behavior in children,[86] and poor executive function has been linked with nonresponse to health interventions in adolescents. A recent study found that executive function moderated the impact of a lifestyle intervention on obese African American adolescents' weight loss, such that adolescents with better executive function participated more and lost more weight than peers with lower executive function.[84] Intriguingly, physical activity benefits on executive function might in turn facilitate increased physical activity, generating greater gains in executive function, and so on, an upward spiral.

Even with limited evidence for efficacy, given the low risk of harm and established health benefits of regular physical activity (eg, physical fitness, weight management, diabetes risk),[58] educators, families, clinicians, and policy makers should integrate physical activity programs into school routines. Participation of overweight and obese youth must be prioritized given the greater health risk in this group, probable greater cognitive benefit, and typical exclusion of such children from athletic programs. T2 translational work is needed to illustrate how best to integrate physical activity into the school day, after school, and other community programs. Programs including Physical Activity Across the Curriculum,[87] Energizers,[88] and Take 10![89] have integrated physical activity with academic lessons, avoiding the competition of physical activity with instructional time.

REFERENCES

1. Ogden CL, Carroll MD, Kit BK, et al. Prevalence of childhood and adult obesity in the United States, 2011-2012. JAMA 2014;311(8):806–14.

2. Skinner AC, Skelton JA. Prevalence and trends in obesity and severe obesity among children in the United States, 1999-2012. JAMA Pediatr 2014;168(6):561–6.

3. Must A, Strauss RS. Risks and consequences of childhood and adolescent obesity. Int J Obes Relat Metab Disord 1999;23(Suppl 2):S2–11.

4. Stroebele N, McNally J, Plog A, et al. The association of self-reported sleep, weight status, and academic performance in fifth-grade students. J Sch Health 2013;83(2):77–84.

5. Rauner A, Mess F, Woll A. The relationship between physical activity, physical fitness and overweight in adolescents: a systematic review of studies published in or after 2000. BMC Pediatr 2013;13:19.

6. Ross N, Yau PL, Convit A. Obesity, fitness, and brain integrity in adolescence. Appetite 2015;93:44–50.

7. Verstynen TD, Weinstein A, Erickson KI, et al. Competing physiological pathways link individual differences in weight and abdominal adiposity to white matter microstructure. Neuroimage 2013;79:129–37.

8. Davis CL, Tkacz JP, Tomporowski PD, et al. Independent associations of organized physical activity and weight status with children's cognitive functioning: a matched-pairs design. Pediatr Exerc Sci 2015;27(4):477–87.

9. Haapala EA, Lintu N, Vaisto J, et al. Associations of physical performance and adiposity with cognition in children. Med Sci Sports Exerc 2015;47(10):2166–74.

10. Li Y, Dai Q, Jackson JC, et al. Overweight is associated with decreased cognitive functioning among school-age children and adolescents. Obesity (Silver Spring) 2008;16(8):1809–15.

11. Tandon P, Thompson S, Moran L, et al. Body mass index mediates the effects of low income on preschool children's executive control, with implications for behavior and academics. Child Obes 2015;11(5):569–76.

12. Wirt T, Schreiber A, Kesztyus D, et al. Early life cognitive abilities and body weight: cross-sectional study of the association of inhibitory control, cognitive flexibility, and sustained attention with BMI percentiles in primary school children. J Obes 2015;2015:534651.

13. Pontifex MB, Kamijo K, Scudder MR, et al. V. The differential association of adiposity and fitness with cognitive control in preadolescent children. Monogr Soc Res Child Dev 2014;79(4):72–92.

14. Datar A, Sturm R, Magnabosco JL. Childhood overweight and academic performance: national study of kindergartners and first-graders. Obes Res 2004;12(1): 58–68.

15. Roberts CK, Freed B, McCarthy WJ. Low fitness and obesity are associated with lower standardized test scores in children. J Pediatr 2010;156(5):711–8.

16. Sardinha LB, Marques A, Martins S, et al. Fitness, fatness, and academic performance in seventh-grade elementary school students. BMC Pediatr 2014;14:176.

17. Torrijos-Nino C, Martinez-Vizcaino V, Pardo-Guijarro MJ, et al. Physical fitness, obesity, and academic achievement in schoolchildren. J Pediatr 2014;165(1): 104–9.

18. Institute of Medicine. Educating the student body: taking physical activity and physical education to school. In: Kohl HW III, Cook HD, editors. Washington, DC: The National Academies Press; 2013. Available at: http://www.iom.edu/Reports/2013/Educating-the-Student-Body-Taking-Physical-Activity-and-Physical-Education-to-School.aspx. Accessed March 3, 2016.

19. Nolan EE, Gadow KD, Sprafkin J. Teacher reports of DSM-IV ADHD, ODD, and CD symptoms in schoolchildren. J Am Acad Child Adolesc Psychiatry 2001; 40(2):241–9.

20. Clotfelter CT, Ladd HF, Vigdor JL. The academic achievement gap in grades 3 to 8. Rev Econ Stat 2009;91(2):398–419.

21. Gordon-Larsen P, Nelson MC, Page P, et al. Inequality in the built environment underlies key health disparities in physical activity and obesity. Pediatrics 2006; 117(2):417–24.

22. Liese AD, D'Agostino RB Jr, Hamman RF, et al. The burden of diabetes mellitus among US youth: prevalence estimates from the SEARCH for diabetes in youth study. Pediatrics 2006;118(4):1510–8.

23. Kramer AF, Hahn S, Cohen NJ, et al. Ageing, fitness and neurocognitive function. Nature 1999;400(6743):418–9.

24. Colcombe SJ, Kramer AF. Fitness effects on the cognitive function of older adults: a meta-analytic study. Psychol Sci 2003;14(2):125–30.

25. Hillman CH, Pontifex MB, Castelli DM, et al. Effects of the FITKids randomized controlled trial on executive control and brain function. Pediatrics 2014;134(4): e1063–71.

26. Kamijo K, Pontifex MB, O'Leary KC, et al. The effects of an afterschool physical activity program on working memory in preadolescent children. Dev Sci 2011; 14(5):1046–58.

27. Chaddock-Heyman L, Erickson KI, Voss MW, et al. The effects of physical activity on functional MRI activation associated with cognitive control in children: a randomized controlled intervention. Front Hum Neurosci 2013;7:72.

28. Kang KD, Choi JW, Kang SG, et al. Sports therapy for attention, cognitions and sociality. Int J Sports Med 2011;32(12):953–9.

29. Hoza B, Smith AL, Shoulberg EK, et al. A randomized trial examining the effects of aerobic physical activity on attention-deficit/hyperactivity disorder symptoms in young children. J Abnorm Child Psychol 2014;43(4):655–67.

30. Choi JW, Han DH, Kang KD, et al. Aerobic exercise and attention deficit hyperactivity disorder: brain research. Med Sci Sports Exerc 2015;47(1):33–9.

31. Reinert KR, Po'e EK, Barkin SL. The relationship between executive function and obesity in children and adolescents: a systematic literature review. J Obes 2013; 2013:820956.

32. Dishman RK, Berthoud HR, Booth FW, et al. Neurobiology of exercise. Obesity (Silver Spring) 2006;14(3):345–56.

33. Buck SM, Hillman CH, Castelli DM. The relation of aerobic fitness to Stroop task performance in preadolescent children. Med Sci Sports Exerc 2008;40(1): 166–72.

34. Hillman CH, Erickson KI, Kramer AF. Be smart, exercise your heart: exercise effects on brain and cognition. Nat Rev Neurosci 2008;9(1):58–65.

35. Davis CL, Cooper S. Fitness, fatness, cognition, behavior, and academic achievement among overweight children: do cross-sectional associations correspond to exercise trial outcomes? Prev Med 2011;52(Suppl 1):S65–9.

36. Diamond A. Executive functions. Annu Rev Psychol 2013;64:135–68.

37. Tomporowski PD, Davis CL, Miller PH, et al. Exercise and children's intelligence, cognition, and academic achievement. Educ Psychol Rev 2008;20(2):111–31. PMC2748863.

38. Davis CL, Tomporowski PD, Boyle CA, et al. Effects of aerobic exercise on overweight children's cognitive functioning: a randomized controlled trial. Res Q Exerc Sport 2007;78(5):510–9.

39. Moher D, Liberati A, Tetzlaff J, et al. Preferred reporting items for systematic reviews and meta-analyses: the PRISMA statement. PLoS Med 2009;6(7): e1000097.

40. Grieco LA, Jowers EM, Bartholomew JB. Physically active academic lessons and time on task: the moderating effect of body mass index. Med Sci Sports Exerc 2009;41(10):1921–6.

41. Tomporowski PD, Davis CL, Lambourne K, et al. Task switching in overweight children: effects of acute exercise and age. J Sport Exerc Psychol 2008;30(5): 497–511.

42. Vazou S, Smiley-Oyen A. Moving and academic learning are not antagonists: acute effects on executive function and enjoyment. J Sport Exerc Psychol 2014;36(5):474–85.

43. Delgado-Rico E, Rio-Valle JS, Albein-Urios N, et al. Effects of a multicomponent behavioral intervention on impulsivity and cognitive deficits in adolescents with excess weight. Behav Pharmacol 2012;23(5–6):609–15.

44. Kinder M, Lotze M, Davids S, et al. Functional imaging in obese children responding to long-term sports therapy. Behav Brain Res 2014;272:25–31.

45. Vanhelst J, Mikulovic J, Hurdiel R, et al. Effects of multidisciplinary program intervention in obese youth on academic performance, sleep, and body composition. Sci Sports 2012;27(3):154–9.

46. Vanhelst J, Marchand F, Fardy P, et al. The CEMHaVi program: control, evaluation, and modification of lifestyles in obese youth. J Cardiopulm Rehabil Prev 2010;30(3):181–5.

47. Kulendran M, Vlaev I, Sugden C, et al. Neuropsychological assessment as a predictor of weight loss in obese adolescents. Int J Obes (Lond) 2014;38(4):507–12.

48. Vanhelst J, Beghin L, Fardy PS, et al. A conative educational model for an intervention program in obese youth. BMC Public Health 2012;12:416.

49. Staiano AE, Abraham AA, Calvert SL. Competitive versus cooperative exergame play for African American adolescents' executive function skills: short-term effects in a long-term training intervention. Dev Psychol 2012;48(2):337–42.

50. Davis CL, Tomporowski PD, McDowell JE, et al. Exercise improves executive function and achievement and alters brain activation in overweight children: a randomized, controlled trial. Health Psychol 2011;30(1):91–8.

51. Crova C, Struzzolino I, Marchetti R, et al. Cognitively challenging physical activity benefits executive function in overweight children. J Sports Sci 2014;32(3): 201–11.

52. Huang T, Larsen KT, Jepsen JR, et al. Effects of an obesity intervention program on cognitive function in children: a randomized controlled trial. Obesity (Silver Spring) 2015;23(10):2101–8.

53. Krafft CE, Pierce JE, Schwarz NF, et al. An eight month randomized controlled exercise intervention alters resting state synchrony in overweight children. Neuroscience 2014;256:445–55.

54. Krafft CE, Schaeffer DJ, Schwarz NF, et al. Improved frontoparietal white matter integrity in overweight children is associated with attendance at an after-school exercise program. Dev Neurosci 2014;36(1):1–9.

55. Krafft CE, Schwarz NF, Chi L, et al. An eight month randomized controlled exercise trial alters brain activation during cognitive tasks in overweight children. Obesity (Silver Spring) 2014;22:232–42.

56. Schaeffer DJ, Krafft CE, Schwarz NF, et al. An 8-month exercise intervention alters frontotemporal white matter integrity in overweight children. Psychophysiology 2014;51(8):728–33.

57. Davis CL, Krafft CE, Waller JL, et al. Cognitive benefits of exercise in overweight children: a randomized controlled trial. Manuscript under review, March 2016.

58. Davis CL, Pollock NK, Waller JL, et al. Exercise dose and diabetes risk in overweight and obese children: a randomized controlled trial. JAMA 2012;308(11): 1103–12.

59. Naglieri JA, Das JP. Cognitive assessment system: interpretive handbook. Itasca (IL): Riverside Publishing; 1997.

60. Diamond A, Lee K. Interventions shown to aid executive function development in children 4 to 12 years old. Science 2011;333(6045):959–64.

61. Best JR. Effects of physical activity on children's executive function: contributions of experimental research on aerobic exercise. Dev Rev 2010;30(4):331–551.

62. Gioia GA, Isquith PK, Guy SC, et al. Behavior rating inventory of executive function. Child Neuropsychol 2000;6(3):235–8.

63. Anderson SE, Economos CD, Must A. Active play and screen time in US children aged 4 to 11 years in relation to sociodemographic and weight status characteristics: a nationally representative cross-sectional analysis. BMC Public Health 2008;8:366.

64. Chang YK, Labban JD, Gapin JI, et al. The effects of acute exercise on cognitive performance: a meta-analysis. Brain Res 2012;1453:87–101.

65. Verburgh L, Konigs M, Scherder EJ, et al. Physical exercise and executive functions in preadolescent children, adolescents and young adults: a meta-analysis. Br J Sports Med 2014;48(12):973–9.

66. Lambourne K, Tomporowski P. The effect of exercise-induced arousal on cognitive task performance: a meta-regression analysis. Brain Res 2010;1341:12–24.

67. Shadish WR, Cook TD, Campbell DT. Experimental and quasi-experimental designs for generalized causal inference. 2nd edition. New York: Houghton Mifflin; 2002.

68. Moher D, Hopewell S, Schulz KF, et al. CONSORT 2010 explanation and elaboration: updated guidelines for reporting parallel group randomised trials. BMJ 2010;340:c869.
69. Bustamante EE, Krafft CE, Schaeffer DJ, et al. The effect of regular exercise on cognition in special populations of children: overweight and attention-deficit hyperactivity disorder. In: McMorris T, editor. Exercise-cognition interaction: neuroscience perspectives. New York: Academic Press, Elsevier; 2016. p. 435-57.
70. Sink KM, Espeland MA, Castro CM, et al. Effect of a 24-month physical activity intervention vs health education on cognitive outcomes in sedentary older adults: the LIFE randomized trial. JAMA 2015;314(8):781-90.
71. Bustamante EE, Davis CL, Frazier SL, et al. Randomized controlled trial of exercise for ADHD and disruptive behavior disorders. Med Sci Sports Exerc 2016. [Epub ahead of print].
72. Schulz KF, Altman DG, Moher D, Consort Group. 2010 statement: updated guidelines for reporting parallel group randomised trials. BMJ 2010;340:c332.
73. Campbell MK, Piaggio G, Elbourne DR, et al. Consort 2010 statement: extension to cluster randomised trials. BMJ 2012;345:e5661.
74. Martin A, Saunders DH, Shenkin SD, et al. Lifestyle intervention for improving school achievement in overweight or obese children and adolescents. Cochrane database Syst Rev 2014;(3):CD009728.
75. Johnston CA, Moreno JP, El-Mubasher A, et al. Impact of a school-based pediatric obesity prevention program facilitated by health professionals. J Sch Health 2013;83(3):171-81.
76. Ahamed Y, Macdonald H, Reed K, et al. School-based physical activity does not compromise children's academic performance. Med Sci Sports Exerc 2007; 39(2):371-6.
77. Winter SM, Sass DA. Healthy & ready to learn: examining the efficacy of an early approach to obesity prevention and school readiness. J Res Child Educ 2011; 25(3):304-25.
78. Flay BR, Biglan A, Boruch RF, et al. Standards of evidence: criteria for efficacy, effectiveness and dissemination. Prev Sci 2005;6(3):151-75.
79. Etnier JL, Nowell PM, Landers DM, et al. A meta-regression to examine the relationship between aerobic fitness and cognitive performance. Brain Res Brain Res Rev 2006;52(1):119-30.
80. Pesce C. Shifting the focus from quantitative to qualitative exercise characteristics in exercise and cognition research. J Sport Exerc Psychol 2012;34(6): 766-86.
81. Kuo FE, Taylor AF. A potential natural treatment for attention-deficit/hyperactivity disorder: evidence from a national study. Am J Public Health 2004;94(9):1580-6.
82. Stranahan AM, Khalil D, Gould E. Social isolation delays the positive effects of running on adult neurogenesis. Nat Neurosci 2006;9(4):526-33.
83. Frazier SL, Chacko A, Van Gessel C, et al. The summer treatment program meets the south side of Chicago: bridging science and service in urban after-school programs. Child Adolesc Ment Health 2012;17(2):86-92.
84. Naar-King S, Ellis DA, Idalski Carcone A, et al. Sequential Multiple Assignment Randomized Trial (SMART) to Construct Weight Loss Interventions for African American Adolescents. J Clin Child Adolesc Psychol 2015. [Epub ahead of print].
85. Buckley J, Cohen JD, Kramer AF, et al. Cognitive control in the self-regulation of physical activity and sedentary behavior. Front Hum Neurosci 2014;8:747.

86. Pentz MA, Riggs NR. Longitudinal relationships of executive cognitive function and parent influence to child substance use and physical activity. Prev Sci 2013;14(3):229–37.

87. Donnelly JE, Greene JL, Gibson CA, et al. Physical activity across the curriculum (PAAC): a randomized controlled trial to promote physical activity and diminish overweight and obesity in elementary school children. Prev Med 2009;49(4): 336–41.

88. Mahar MT, Murphy SK, Rowe DA, et al. Effects of a classroom-based program on physical activity and on-task behavior. Med Sci Sports Exerc 2006;38(12): 2086–94.

89. Kibbe DL, Hackett J, Hurley M, et al. Ten years of TAKE 10!: integrating physical activity with academic concepts in elementary school classrooms. Prev Med 2011;52(Suppl 1):S43–50.

Treating Obesity in Preschoolers

A Review and Recommendations for Addressing Critical Gaps

Elizabeth K. Towner, PhD[a],*, Lisa M. Clifford, PhD[b],
Mary Beth McCullough, PhD[c], Cathleen Odar Stough, PhD[c],
Lori J. Stark, PhD[d]

KEYWORDS

- Preschool • Obesity • Intervention

KEY POINTS

- Nearly one-quarter of preschoolers are overweight or obese, with persistent disparities among those from low-income and minority backgrounds.
- Developing interventions effective at obesity reduction in early childhood is imperative given the immediate physical and psychosocial health consequences of excess weight gain and its persistence to adulthood if not addressed.
- Poor reach to families from low-income and minority backgrounds, insufficient evidence to determine the most effective and efficient treatment components and approaches to treating obesity in early childhood, and lack of consensus on how best to discern intervention effectiveness are 3 critical gaps in the preschool obesity treatment literature.
- Addressing these gaps is imperative to eliminating preschool obesity disparities and reducing the overall prevalence of obesity in early childhood.

Disclosure Statement: This review was supported by grants R21HD078890 (E.K. T) and T32DK063929 (Scott Powers) from the National Institutes of Health.
[a] Department of Family Medicine and Public Health Sciences, Wayne State University School of Medicine, Wayne State University, IBio 6135 Woodward Avenue, H206, Detroit, MI 48202, USA; [b] Department of Clinical and Health Psychology, College of Public Health & Health Professions, University of Florida, P.O. Box 100165, Gainesville, FL 32610-0165, USA; [c] Division of Behavioral Medicine & Clinical Psychology, Cincinnati Children's Hospital Medical Center, MLC 7039, 3333 Burnet Avenue, Cincinnati, OH 45229-3039, USA; [d] Division of Behavioral Medicine & Clinical Psychology, Cincinnati Children's Hospital Medical Center, MLC 3015, 3333 Burnet Avenue, Cincinnati, OH 45229-3039, USA
* Corresponding author.
E-mail address: ekuhl@med.wayne.edu

Pediatr Clin N Am 63 (2016) 481–510
http://dx.doi.org/10.1016/j.pcl.2016.02.005
0031-3955/16/$ – see front matter © 2016 Elsevier Inc. All rights reserved.

INTRODUCTION

Twenty-three percent of 2- to 5-year-old children in the United States are estimated to be overweight (body mass index [BMI] ≥85th percentile) or obese (BMI ≥95th percentile).[1] Although rates have decreased over the last decade, these changes have not been experienced equally, and disparities persist for preschoolers from low-income and minority backgrounds.[1,2] Excess weight gain in early childhood remains a significant public health concern given immediate physical and psychosocial health consequences (eg, high blood pressure, run/walk difficulties, peer stigmatization, lower health-related quality of life),[3–6] its persistence into adolescence and adulthood,[7–9] and the implications for morbidity and mortality in adulthood even when controlling for adult weight status.[10] Early intervention (before age 6) is important because the incidence of new-onset obesity is greater during kindergarten than any other time in childhood,[11] because children overweight at kindergarten are 4 times more likely to become obese later in childhood,[11] and because prevention efforts have unclear benefits for preschoolers who already overweight and obese.[12–14]

A recent comprehensive review of the preschool obesity intervention literature by Foster and colleagues[15] concluded multidisciplinary, intensive behavioral programs seem most promising for achieving the goal of obesity reduction in children younger than 6 years. This report moves beyond examining efficacy to explore the current state of the preschool obesity treatment literature by critically evaluating the sociodemographic reach of preschool obesity interventions (ie, who is enrolling), which lifestyle behaviors and behavior change strategies are most efficient and effective for yielding improvements in preschooler weight status, and how to best evaluate program effectiveness. Integrated into this discussion is a call to focus on early-stage intervention development to address critical gaps in each of these domains and to concentrate efforts on developing interventions for families from low-income and minority backgrounds. The same criteria for intervention inclusion used by Foster and colleagues[15] were applied for this review: (1) enrolled children ages 0 to 6 years (or tailoring to preschoolers if sample included older children), (2) included measure of weight status, and (3) only included children with BMI ≥85th percentile. We identified one additional publication beyond Foster and colleagues,[15,16] bringing the total number of studies included in this review to 7.

Reach of Preschool Weight Control Trials

Preschool obesity interventions should be designed to maximize reach so eligible families are aware of the intervention and participate.[17] Understanding enrollment rates, sociodemographic characteristics of who is enrolling, which strategies are most effective in recruiting families, and barriers (eg, transportation, perception of health problem) to participation are important first steps in evaluating the progress of the preschool obesity treatment literature. Here each trial is evaluated to discern answers to these questions. Recruitment details and characteristics of intervention arms are summarized by trial and detailed in **Tables 1** and **2**.

Two trials were conducted within established pediatric obesity clinics to which participants had already been referred by a pediatrician or health care provider and agreed to receive treatment.[18,19] Both trials were conducted outside of the United States, and neither provided information on sociodemographic characteristics of participating families. In the first study by Bocca and colleagues,[18] all but 3 referred families met eligibility criteria and were randomly assigned to receive either a 4-month, 25-session multidisciplinary program or usual care. In the second study by Kelishadi and colleagues,[19] all 120 referred families enrolled and were randomly assigned to one of three 6-month, 6-session interventions: energy restriction, dairy rich, or education only (control).

Table 1
Recruitment and sample characteristics

Study	Number Attempted/ Invited	Number Eligible	Number (%) of Eligible Enrolled	Sample Characteristics, M± SSB/n (%)
Kelishadi et al,[19] 2009	120	120	120 (100%)	Child Age[a]: 5.6 ± 0.5 BMI SSBS: Dairy-rich diet = 2.4 ± 0.01 Energy-restricted diet = 2.3 ± 0.04 Control = 2.4 ± 0.01 BMI: Dairy-rich diet = 22.1 ± 0.09 Energy-restricted diet = 22.7 ± 0.8 Control = 22.4 ± 0.5
Stark et al,[20] 2011	109	56	18 (32%)	Child BMI Percentile: Intervention = 99 ± 0.9 ESC = 97.7 ± 2.5 Age: Intervention = 4.4 ± 0.92 ESC = 3.9 ± 1.1 Sex (female): Intervention = 2 (25) ESC = 4 (40) Minority: Intervention = 3 (25) ESC = 1 (10) Hispanic: Intervention = 2 (25) ESC = 1 (10) Caregiver[b] Age: Intervention = 36 ± 3.61 ESC = 35 ± 4.24 Education (≥college degree): Intervention = 5 (62.5) ESC = 6 (60) Income (≥$50,000 annually): Intervention = 8 (100) ESC = 8 (80)
Taveras et al,[23] 2011	3253	1008	475 (47%)	Child Age: Intervention = 4.8 ± 1.2 Usual Care = 5.2 ± 1.1 Minority: Intervention = 135 (53) Usual care = 58 (30) BMI z-score: Intervention = 1.88 ± 0.69 Usual care = 1.82 ± 0.56 BMI: Intervention = 19.2 ± 2.6 Usual Care = 19.2 ± 2.0 Caregiver Obese: Intervention = 154 (61) Usual care = 84 (44) Education (>college): Intervention = 147 (58)

(continued on next page)

Study	Number Attempted/ Invited	Number Eligible	Number (%) of Eligible Enrolled	Sample Characteristics, M± SSB/n (%)
				Usual care = 127 (66)
				Income (≥$50,000 annually):
				Intervention = 160 (64)
				Usual care = 153 (80)
				Marital status (married):
				Intervention = 187 (75)
				Usual care = 151 (79)
Bocca et al,[18] 2012; Bocca et al,[114] 2014	78	75	75 (100%)	Child
				Age:
				Intervention = 4.6 ± 0.8
				Usual care = 4.7 ± 0.8
				Sex (female):
				Intervention = 28 (70)
				Usual care = 12 (30)
				BMI:
				Intervention = 21.2 ± 2.9
				Usual care = 21.0 ± 2.7
				BMI z-score:
				Intervention = 2.7 ± 1.0
				Usual care = 2.7 ± 1.0
Quattrin et al,[21] 2012; Quattrin et al,[22] 2014	171	147	105 (71%)	Child
				Age:
				Intervention = 4.6 ± 1.1
				Control = 4.4 ± 1.1
				Sex (female):
				Intervention = 31 (67)
				Control = 33 (66)
				Minority:
				Intervention = 13 (28)
				Control = 13 (26)
				BMI z-score:
				Intervention = 2.2 ± 0.8
				Control = 2.1 ± 0.7
				% Over BMI:
				Intervention = 32.4 ± 22.4
				Control = 29.8 ± 17.1
				Caregiver
				Age:
				Intervention = 37.2 ± 5.0
				Control = 36.4 ± 5.0
				Sex (female):
				Intervention = 33 (72)
				Control = 39 (78)
				Minority:
				Intervention = 12 (26)
				Control = 8 (16)
				Income:
				Median = $65,729
				<$20,000 = 8 (8.3)
				BMI:
				Intervention = 37.2 ± 8.3
				Control = 36.2 ± 6.9

(continued on next page)

	Number		Number (%)	
	Attempted/	Number	of Eligible	
Study	Invited	Eligible	Enrolled	Sample Characteristics, M± SSB/n (%)
van Grieken et al,[24] 2013	13792[c]	unknown	637[d]	**Child**
				Age (mo):
				Intervention = 68.65 ± 4.98
				Control = 69.64 ± 5.37
				Sex (female):
				Intervention = 214 (61.3)
				Control = 179 (62.3)
				Minority:
				Intervention = 80 (24.2)
				Control = 56 (19.4)
				BMI:
				Intervention = 18.6 ± 0.63
				Control = 18.10 ± 0.61
				Mothers
				Age:
				Intervention = 35.8 ± 4.23
				Control = 35.92 ± 4.37
				Education (mid-high/high):
				Intervention = 333 (66.7)
				Control = 197 (68.5)
				BMI (overweight/obese)
				Intervention = 155 (44.5)
				Control = 135 (43.4)
Stark et al,[16] 2014	277	153	42 (27%)	**Child**
				Age:
				ESC = 4.8 ± 0.7
				IHV = 4.7 ± 1.3
				ICO = 4.2 ± 1.1
				Sex (female):
				ESC = 8 (67)
				IHV = 8 (80)
				ICO = 7 (64)
				Minority:
				ESC = 3 (25)
				IHV = 1 (10)
				ICO = 1 (9)
				BMIz:
				ESC = 2.4 ± 0.4
				IHV = −2.1 ± 2.1
				ICO = 2.5 ± 2.5
				Family Income (≥$50,000 annually):
				ESC = 10 (83)
				IHV = 8 (99)
				ICO = 9 (82)

Abbreviations: ESC, enhanced standard of care; ICO, intervention clinic only; IHV, Intervention with home visits.

[a] Age only reported in the report for sample as a whole.

[b] Sample characteristics are for mothers only, as few fathers were primary caregivers targeted for intervention (Mothers, 7 [87.5%]; Control, 9 [90%]).

[c] Number reflects all families invited, as recruitment information was not presented by preschooler weight status.

[d] Percentage of enrollment cannot be determined because recruitment flow was not differentiated by preschooler weight status.

Table 2
Preschool weight control trial characteristics

Study	Trial Arm	Length	Dose	Session Location	Session Length	Interventionist(s)	Format
Kelishadi et al,[19] 2009	Healthy lifestyle education + dairy rich	6 mo	6 monthly	Obesity research center	Did not report	Pediatrician and nutritionist	Group
	Healthy lifestyle education + energy restriction	6 mo	6 monthly sessions	Obesity research center	Did not report	Pediatrician and nutritionist	Group
	Healthy lifestyle education (control)	6 mo	6 monthly sessions	Obesity research center	Did not report	Pediatrician and nutritionist	Group
Stark et al,[20] 2011	Intervention	6 mo	18 sessions (weekly for 3 mo, biweekly for 3 mo)	Academic medical center and homes of participating families	90-min group sessions, 60–90 min home visits	PhD-level psychologist (parent groups); pediatric psychology postdoctoral fellow and research coordinator (child groups); pediatric psychology postdoctoral fellow (home visits)	Group and Individual
	Control-Enhanced standard of care	1 session	1 session	Academic medical center (≤50 miles from homes of participating families)	45–60 min sessions	Pediatrician	Individual
Taveras et al,[23] 2011	Intervention	1 y	4 in-person sessions and 3 phone calls	Pediatrician's office	25-min in-person sessions and 15-minute phone sessions	Pediatric nurse practitioners	Individual families
	Usual care	1 y	1 well-child visit	Pediatrician's office	Did not specify	Pediatricians	Individual families

Study	Arm	Duration	Sessions	Setting	Session length	Provider	Format
Bocca et al,[18] 2012; Bocca et al,[114] 2014	Intervention	4 mo	25 sessions (behavioral therapy: 6 sessions; PA: 12 sessions; dietary advice: 6 sessions)	Groningen Expert Center for Kids with Obesity	(behavioral therapy sessions: 30–120 min; PA sessions: 60 min; dietary advice: 30 min)	Psychologist, physiotherapist Registered dietician	Group
	Control	4 mo	3 sessions	Groningen Expert Center for Kids with Obesity	30–60 min sessions	Pediatrician	Group
Quattrin et al,[21] 2012; Quattrin et al,[22] 2014	Intervention	6 mo	10 sessions (4 weekly, 2 bimonthly, 4 monthly); 8 phone calls in between meetings	Primary care	60-min sessions	Patient enhancement assistants and project manager = group leaders; pediatricians reviewed progress at 3 and 6 mo	Group
	Information control	6 mo	10 sessions (4 weekly, 2 bimonthly, 4 monthly); 8 phone calls in between meetings	Primary care	60-min sessions	Group leaders trained to deliver intervention; pediatricians reviewed progress at 3 and 6 mo	Group
van Grieken et al,[24] 2013	Intervention	1 y	Up to 4 sessions	Youth health care centers	Did not specify	Physician-nurse teams, mostly physicians	Individual
	Usual care control	1 y	1 session	Youth health care centers	Did not specify	Physician-nurse teams, mostly Physicians	Individual

(continued on next page)

Table 2
(continued)

Study	Trial Arm	Length	Dose	Session Location	Session Length	Interventionist(s)	Format
Stark et al,[16] 2014	Intervention-clinic and home	6 mo	18 sessions (weekly for 3 mo, biweekly for 3 mo)	Academic medical center (≤50 miles from homes of participating families) and homes of participating families	90-min group sessions, 60–90 min home visits	PhD-level psychologist (parent groups); pediatric psychology postdoctoral fellow and research coordinator (child groups); pediatric psychology postdoctoral fellow (home visits)	Group and Individual
	Intervention-clinic only	6 mo	9 sessions (biweekly for 3 mo, monthly for 3 mo)	Academic medical center as control (≤50 miles from homes of participating families)	90 min sessions	PhD-level psychologist (parent groups); pediatric psychology postdoctoral fellow and research coordinator (child groups)	Group
	Control-Enhanced standard of care	1 session	1 session	Academic medical center	45–60 min sessions	Pediatrician	Individual

Three trials examined intensive behavioral interventions[16,20,21]; all required one caregiver who was overweight for participation. Two iterative pilot randomized, controlled trials by Stark and colleagues[16,20] examined the efficacy of a 6-month, 18-session clinic and home-based intervention targeting obesity reduction in preschoolers and caregivers compared with an enhanced standard-of-care session with a pediatrician. Clinic visits were group based. The second iteration[16] also included a third intervention arm (9 sessions, clinic-only program). Prescreened families of preschoolers with obesity were randomly selected to receive a study invitation letter and opt-out postcard from their pediatrician. The research team called all families who did not return opt-out postcards within 10 days of the mailings. Across the trials, 51% of families reached refused participation. Twenty-six percent of eligible families enrolled, of which, 18% were from minority backgrounds, and 16% reported an annual income ≤$50,000 (the lowest income bracket assessed). Quattrin and colleagues[21,22] tested an intensive behavioral intervention (12 months, 13 in-person sessions plus 10 coaching calls between group visits) delivered within a primary care setting. Families were randomized to an intervention or control group. Only the program for intervention families included behavior modification and child management skills training and targeted weight management for preschoolers and caregivers. Study recruiters were embedded within the primary care clinic and met with interested families immediately after well-child visits. Twenty-five percent of families referred by pediatricians declined to meet with recruiters. Eighty-one percent of eligible families enrolled in the trial, of which, 26% were from minority backgrounds and 8.3% reported an annual income of ≤20,000 (the lowest income bracket assessed).

In 2 trials, randomization occurred at the clinic or provider level. Interventions tested were less intensive (≤10 sessions over a year) and occurred within the primary care setting.[23,24] Taveras and colleagues[23] randomly assigned pediatrician offices to deliver a 1-year program consisting of 4 office visits and 3 phone calls (intervention) or continue with usual care. An invitation letter opt-out procedure like that of Stark and colleagues[16,20] was used for recruitment. Twenty-one percent of families contacted by phone declined participation. Forty-seven percent of eligible families enrolled, of which, 43% of families were from minority backgrounds and 29% reported an annual income of ≤$50,000 (the lowest income bracket assessed in the study). In the second trial, van Grieken and colleagues[24] randomly assigned Youth Health Care teams within 9 Youth Health Care Centers to provide a 12-month, ≤4-session motivational interviewing plus counseling intervention, or usual care to families of 5-year-old overweight preschoolers. Rates of refusal, the total number of eligible families, and sociodemographic characteristics for families with overweight preschoolers are unclear, as study participation was offered to families irrespective of child weight, and recruitment flow was not presented by preschooler weight status. A total of 637 families with overweight preschoolers enrolled.

In summary, rates of enrollment (26%–81%) and refusal (21%–51%) into preschool weight control trials are variable. However, low representation of families from low-income (8.3%–29%) and minority (18%–43%) backgrounds is more consistent (see **Table 1**). This finding is concerning given the persistence of obesity disparities. Only 2 studies provided information on barriers to participation. Although interventions differed in intensity and structure, time (61–66%) and not believing preschooler weight is problematic (27–29%) were the most frequently cited barriers to enrollment by families who were contacted about trial participation.[20,25] Although Taveras and colleagues[25] found lower enrollment for families with more highly educated caregivers, they did not evaluate whether income or race/ethnicity differentiated families who refused participation. All trials recruited families from medical settings. Excluding the 2 trials in which families had accessed services in a weight management clinic before being invited to participate in research,[18,19] enrollment was highest when recruitment was initiated by pediatricians, occurred entirely in person, and when interventions were implemented within the primary care settings.[21,23,24]

Future directions to improve reach

First, caregivers from LIAA backgrounds often have inaccurate perceptions of preschooler weight status and lack concern about preschooler excess weight gain.[4–7] As such, they may be less motivated to participate in obesity interventions. Based on limitations described, 3 recommendations are provided to improve reach of preschool obesity interventions. First, strategies are needed to increase the accuracy of caregiver perceptions of child weight status and their motivation for change, particularly among families from low-income and minority backgrounds.[26–29] Inaccuracy may also reflect that pediatricians are less likely to talk about weight or diagnose obesity in preschoolers compared with older pediatric age groups.[30,31] Color-coded BMI charts are one tool that has effectively facilitated more frequent weight discussions with pediatricians and improved caregiver accuracy in perception of child weight status, particularly among families of preschoolers from low-income and minority backgrounds.[32–34] Dawson and colleagues[34] also found 76% of families who received weight feedback using color-coded BMI charts enrolled into a 2-year preschool weight control trial in New Zealand. Culturally tailored weight rulers are an additional tool that shows promise in improving accuracy of caregiver perceptions of preschooler weight status and were preferred over color-coded BMI charts by families from low-income and minority backgrounds.[35]

Second, expanding recruitment beyond medical settings may improve enrollment of families from low-income and minority backgrounds. Emergency departments are one setting that could be explored for its recruitment potential given their frequent use by low-income and minority populations for routine health care.[36,37] Further, Lynch and colleagues[38] recently found significantly higher emergency department use by overweight and obese children compared with those who were of a healthy weight. Researchers should also establish partnerships with The Special Supplemental Nutrition Program for Women, Infants, and Children (WIC) and Head Start, as these federally funded programs serve 4.7[39] and 1 million[40] preschoolers from low-income backgrounds, respectively. Further, more than 40% of families receiving services from WIC and Head Start are from racial and ethnic minority backgrounds. Preschool obesity trials are currently underway that may provide insight on the recruitment potential of collaborating with these community-based organizations.[41,42] Finally, YMCAs should be considered given their general emphasis on health promotion and because pediatric weight control programs have been successfully implemented in this setting.[43]

Third, even if caregiver motivation increases and recruitment is extended beyond medical settings, families may still be reluctant to enroll in preschool weight control trials if they do not perceive the intervention as feasible and acceptable. As noted previously, a substantial number of families contacted by Stark and colleagues[20] and Taveras and colleagues[23] reported time as a barrier to enrollment. Interventions tested in each study varied on intensity, dose, and treatment setting, which suggests additional intervention characteristics other than time may serve as enrollment barriers (see **Table 2**). Ongoing trials may provide insight on whether innovative components improve enrollment, especially among low-income and minority populations. For example, 3 studies are testing programs led by community health workers,[41,42,44] and 2 of these studies are entirely home based.[42,44] Examining enrollment characteristics de novo can provide information on feasibility and acceptability but may slow progress and is costly because trials must be completed before analysis. Recently, the Obesity-Related Behavioral Intervention Trials (ORBIT) work group published a 4-phase model for developing health behavioral interventions[45] that encourages completion of 2 formative phases before conducting comparative effectiveness trials. Involving members of the targeted population from the start of program development (user-centered approach) is encouraged to maximize intervention feasibility and acceptability. Only one trial,[41] which is currently underway, involved their target population (WIC families) in the formative steps of intervention development. Specifically, semistructured qualitative interviews were completed with families of overweight and obese preschoolers to discern why they felt it was important to address weight in early childhood and the feasibility and acceptability of extent preschool obesity interventions.[46] Information gleaned from interviews was applied to develop the 4-month (14 session), community- and home-based preschool weight control intervention that is currently being pilot tested.[41] A full example of how the National Institutes of Health ORBIT model can be applied to complete the formative steps of developing interventions for low-income and minority populations via increasing feasibility and acceptability is presented in **Tables 3** and **4**.

Treatment Components

Identifying which lifestyle behaviors or combination of behaviors are most salient to reducing obesity in preschool-age children and how to best help families achieve these behavior changes is a second important step to advancing the preschool obesity treatment literature. This section reviews what is currently known about lifestyle behaviors contributing to excess weight gain in early childhood (eg, diet, activity, sleep), the unique challenges to modifying these behaviors for preschoolers, and evidence for what strategies are effective in changing behaviors associated with increased obesity risk in early childhood. **Table 5** provides an overview of behaviors targeted, specific recommendations, if and how behavior change was measured, and changes reported within the 7 published preschool weight control trials.

Diet

Preschoolers are estimated to consume an average of 1537 calories daily,[47] which exceeds the 1000 to 1400 calories recommended for moderately active children based on age and sex.[48] Palatable foods like pasta, desserts, milk (whole and reduced fat), and fruit juice are the largest contributors to daily caloric intake for preschoolers,[49] with slightly less than half meeting daily fruit and vegetable (FV) recommendations.[50] Sugar sweetened beverages (SSBs, eg, soda, fruit drinks) and snacks are estimated to account for approximately 10%[49] and 27%[51] of preschoolers' daily caloric intake, respectively. Although caregivers of preschoolers have more control over their child's dietary intake than perhaps at any other developmental period, normative preschool behaviors present a challenge to dietary modification. Because children innately prefer salty and sweet tastes,[52] foods that do not have these properties (eg, vegetables) are often rejected.[53] Food neophobia, the rejection of novel or unknown foods,[54] peaks during the preschool years.[55] Tantrumming for food is also commonly reported by caregivers of preschoolers and associated with increased obesity risk.[56] Caregivers frequently discontinue exposure to new foods after 3 to 5 trials[57] instead of the 12 to 15 necessary for new food preferences to develop.[58] Caregivers of preschoolers also report frequently using food to manage child behaviors by providing palatable foods as rewards for good behavior and to terminate disruptive behaviors.[59–61]

Table 3
Example of how to apply the National Institutes of Health ORBIT model to complete formative steps of developing a preschool obesity intervention for underserved populations

Phase	Example
1: Design	
1a: Define	• Review guidelines and empirical literature to identify promising behavioral targets, change strategies, and intervention approaches/structure • Semistructured qualitative interviews or focus groups with targeted population to complete needs assessment and determine feasibility and acceptability of extant interventions
1b: Refine	• Semistructured qualitative interviews or focus groups with targeted population provide feedback on content, structure, dose, delivery setting/method of beta version of intervention developed from information collected in "define" stage • Ideally would include having members of the targeted population complete a particular session or utilize a specific strategy (eg, new self-monitoring tool) for a shortened period • Adapt and modifying intervention based on feedback from participants
2: Preliminary testing	
2a: Proof-of-concept	• Open trial (small number) in which members of the targeted population complete the intervention • Include qualitative methodology to gather in-depth feedback from families on their intervention experience. • If possible, and needed, complete interviews with families who drop out to understand what (if anything) could be done differently to promote retention. • Adapt and modify intervention based on feedback from participants and outcome data. • Repeat until intervention achieves clinically significant reduction in preschooler obesity status.
2b: Pilot studies	• Pilot randomized, controlled trial with adequate control group (eg, treatment as usual in primary care or WIC). • Include qualitative methodology to gather information on intervention feasibility and acceptability with all or randomly selected subset of intervention completers. • If possible, and needed, complete interviews with families who drop out to understand what (if anything) could be done differently to promote retention. • Adapt and modify intervention as warranted based on feedback from participants and outcome data. • Repeat until intervention achieves significantly greater reduction in preschooler obesity status compared with the control condition.

From Czajkowski SM, Powell LH, Adler N, et al. From ideas to efficacy: the ORBIT model for developing behavioral treatments for chronic diseases. Health Psychol 2015;34(10):971–82.

Managing negative food-related behaviors seems especially challenging for caregivers of preschoolers who are overweight and obese, as they report uncertainty in how to encourage consumption of new foods, feeling like they are depriving children if unhealthy foods are limited, and difficulty managing tantrums resulting from restricting access to unhealthy foods.[62,63] Strategies caregivers use to encourage healthy eating may also have the opposite of their intended effect. For example, restricting access to highly palatable foods is associated with greater intake of those foods when accessible, even in the absence of hunger,[64] and higher weight.[64–66] Similarly,

Table 4	
Barriers and recommendations for improving reach of preschool obesity interventions	
Barrier/Challenge	**Recommendation**
Inaccurate perception of child weight status	• Increased discussion of weight with pediatrician • Increased frequency of diagnosing overweight and obesity by pediatrician • Use of tools to increase accuracy of caregiver perception of child weight status (eg, weight rulers and color-coded BMI charts)
Recruitment limited to medical settings (weight management clinics and pediatrician offices)	• Expand recruitment to other settings frequented by families with overweight and obese children such as the emergency department • Partner with community organizations, especially those serving predominately low-income and minority families
Failure to include families of overweight and obese preschoolers in the treatment development process	• Formative studies to explore with families of obese preschoolers what they want and need in programs targeting obesity reduction • Emphasis on understanding needs of families from low-income and minority backgrounds given these populations are underrepresented in the preschool obesity treatment literature despite being at greater obesity risk

pressuring children to eat certain foods (eg, vegetables), is associated with decreased preference for those foods,[67] and picky eating.[68–70]

In light of these patterns and challenges, it is not surprising dietary modification is a component of all preschool weight control interventions included in this review. However, there is significant variability in which behaviors are targeted and how (see **Table 5**). Decreasing caloric intake is the most common dietary recommendation. Four[16,18–20] of 5[16,18–21] studies including this component report outcome data. Although caloric intake decreased for intervention preschoolers in all 4 studies, this change was only significantly greater than controls or alternate treatments in studies by Stark and colleagues.[16,20] Stark and colleagues[16,20] also document the only maintenance of caloric decreases achieved during intervention participation at a 6-month follow-up assessment. Decreasing SSB intake increasing and FV intake are the second most common dietary targets.[16,20,21,23] Outcome data were reported for 2[23,71] of 3[21,23,71] interventions including recommendations for one or both of these behavior changes. Taveras and colleagues[23] found modest decreases in SSBs and increases in FV for preschoolers irrespective of group assignment, but neither group achieved the recommended amount. Kuhl and colleagues[71] collapsed data for 2 iterative trials of a clinic- and home-based behavioral intervention. Intervention preschoolers experienced a small and nonsignificant decrease in SSB that was consistent with recommendations. FV intake increased significantly but not to recommended levels. Only Taveras and colleagues[23] specifically targeted fast food consumption, finding marginally larger changes for preschoolers in the intervention compared with the control group. Additional dietary targets for which no outcome data were reported include eating breakfast daily,[24] portion control,[21,24] and limiting snacking.[24] Across the 7 trials, only Kuhl and colleagues[71] specifically examined the relationship between dietary changes (calories, FVs, SSB, sweet and salty snacks) and weight outcomes, finding that decreases in caloric intake was the only significant dietary predictor of BMI z-score (BMIz) reductions for intervention preschoolers.

Table 5
Summary of components and behavior change data

Study	Behaviors Targeted	Recommendation/ Daily Goal	How Change Measured	ΔBaseline posttreatment	ΔBaseline to 12 mo[a]
Kelishadi et al,[19] 2009	Caloric intake	NS	Diary (3 d)	MNR	MNR
	Calcium intake	NS	Diary (3 d)	MNR	MNR
	Activity	NS	Parent report	MNR	MNR
Stark et al,[20] 2011	Caloric intake	1000–1400[b]	24-h dietary recalls	LHV = −218 ± 354 ESC = 322 ± 280	LHV = −214 ± 327 ESC = 311 ± 372
	FVs	5 servings	24-h dietary recalls	NR[c]	NR[c]
	MVPA	60 min	Accelerometer	NR[c]	NR[c]
	Screen use	≤2 h	Parent report	NR[c]	NR[c]
	SSBs	Reduce/eliminate	24-h dietary recalls	NR[c]	NR[c]
Taveras et al,[23] 2011	SSBs	<4 ounces	Parent report	I = −0.59 ± 0.10 C = −0.33 ± 0.06	N/A
	Fast food	≤1 outing per wk	Parent report	I = −0.22 ± 0.05 C = −0.02 ± 0.06	
	Screen use	≤1 h	Parent report	I = −0.53 ± 0.09 C = −0.07 ± 0.09	
	Television in bedroom	Remove	Parent report	I = −25(10%) C = −9(5%)	
	FV	5 servings	Parent report	I = 0.22 ± 0.09 C = 0.16 ± 0.11	
	Outdoor active playtime	60≥ min	Parent report	I = 0.06 ± 0.10 C = 0.20 ± 0.13	
Bocca et al,[18] 2012; Bocca et al,[114] 2014	Caloric intake[d]	Normocalorie diet	Diet diary	$I_{Baseline}$ = 1434 ± 252 $I_{Posttreatment}$ = 1323 ± 200 $C_{Baseline}$ = 1504 ± 316 $C_{Posttreatment}$ = 1327 ± 220	$I_{Follow-up}$ = 1369 ± 244 $C_{Follow-up}$ = 1429 ± 265
	Activity[d]	60 min	Pedometer (step count)	$I_{Baseline}$ = 11,998 ± 3031 $I_{Posttreatment}$ = 13,823 ± 2711 $C_{Baseline}$ = 9862 ± 2729 $C_{Posttreatment}$ = 1327 ± 220	$I_{Follow-up}$ = 12,455 ± 3185 $C_{Follow-up}$ = 1429 ± 265

Study	Behavior	Target	Measurement	I	C
Quattrin et al,[21] 2012; Quattrin et al,[22] 2014	Caloric intake	1000–1400[b]	Diary	NR	NR
	Activity	60 min	Diary	NR	NR
	TV/screen time	<2 h	Diary	NR	NR
van Grieken et al,[24] 2013	Playing outdoors	1 ≥ h daily	NA	NR	NR
	Eating breakfast	<2 glasses	NA	NR	NR
	SSBs	Reduce	NA	NR	NR
	Screen activity	Reduce	NA	NR	NR
Stark et al,[16] 2014	Caloric intake	1000–1400[b]	24-h dietary recalls	LHV = -465 ± 292 LC = -243 ± 567 ESC = -65 ± 724	LHV = -518 ± 315 LC = -249 ± 592 ESC = 3 ± 620
	FVs	5 servings	24-h dietary recalls	NR[c]	NR[c]
	MVPA	60 min	Accelerometer	NR[c]	NR[c]
	Screen use	≤2 h	Parent report	NR[c]	NR[c]
	SSBs	Reduce/eliminate	24-h dietary recalls	NR[c]	NR[c]
Kuhl et al,[71] 2014	Caloric intake	1000–1400[b]	24-h dietary recalls	LHV = -72.48 ± 351.93	N/A
	FVs	5 servings	24-h dietary recalls	LHV = 1.16 ± 3.03	
	MVPA	60 min	Accelerometer	LHV = 4.37 ± 18.13	
	Screen use	≤2 h	Parent report	LHV = -26.96 ± 69.34	
	SSBs	Reduce/eliminate	24-h dietary recalls	LHV = -1.82 ± 4.22	

Abbreviations: C, control; ESC, enhanced standard of care; FVs, fruits and vegetables; I, intervention; LC, LAUNCH clinic only; LHV, LAUNCH Home Visits; MNR, means not reported (data available only in graphical form); MVPA, moderate-to-vigorous physical activity; NR, not reported; NS, not specified; SSBs, sugar sweetened beverages.

a Although 3 studies included follow-up assessments at 1 up to 3 years posttreatment, outcome data on behavior changes were either not reported[22,114] or means could not be discerned from graphs.[19]

b Daily calorie recommendations based on preschooler age and sex: 2 to 3 years old, 1000; 4- to 6-year-old girls, 1200; 4- to 6-year-old boys, 1400.

c Outcomes for preschoolers randomly assigned to LHV collapsed across iterative trials and reported in Kuhl and colleagues.[71]

d Change scores not reported.

Strategies taught for achieving dietary changes include self-monitoring,[16,18,20,21,23,24] shaping,[16,20,21] stimulus control,[16,20,21] modeling,[16,20,21] an interactive Web site with recipes,[23] vegetable taste tests,[16,20] positive feeding practices,[16,20] and child behavior management strategies.[16,20,21,24] However, data on participant use of these strategies and the relationship between strategy implementation and behavior changes is lacking. Stark and colleagues[16,20] provide the only outcome data on use of behavior change strategies, and this report is limited to stimulus control within the home food environment. Providing education and engaging families in "home clean-outs" at home visits yielded significantly greater reductions in high-calorie foods for families in the intervention compared with control groups that were maintained to the 6-month follow-up. Although significantly greater increases in FVs and decreases in SSBs were evident for intervention compared with control families at posttreatment, changes were not sustained at the 6-month follow-up.

Physical activity Similar to diet, unique challenges to modifying physical activity (PA) are evident during the preschool years. Unlike older pediatric age groups and adults, preschoolers are physically active in isolated and sporadic spurts[72,73] that can range from a fraction of a second to 9 minutes.[74] Because only a small portion of activity spurts reach the moderate-to-vigorous activity level, it can take more than 11 hours for preschoolers to meet the recommended 60 minutes of daily moderate-to-vigorous PA (MVPA).[74] Parent-reported barriers to increasing preschooler PA include lack of knowledge about what constitutes MVPA, difficulty measuring daily activity, outdoor safety, inability to monitor or engage in PA with their child, parent dislike of PA, and inclement weather.[75,76] Caregivers may overestimate the amount of PA their preschoolers are getting at (pre)school or daycare,[77] which may further hinder encouraging PA at home. Although homes of obese preschoolers are found to have fewer PA devices,[78,79] studies have not consistently found preschoolers who are overweight or obese to engage in lower levels of PA than their healthy-weight peers.[80] However, an inverse association between vigorous PA and being overweight in preschoolers has been found.[81]

Although PA was included as a component within all published preschool obesity interventions, the type of activity targeted varied. Stark and colleagues[16,20] found MVPA remained stable and consistent with recommendations across all assessment time points with no differences for preschoolers in the intervention compared to control conditions. Although all preschoolers in the trial conducted by Bocca and colleagues[18] increased their daily step count, increases were only significant for those in the control condition, and there were no between-group differences. Kelishadi and colleagues[19] reported energy expenditure increases (not significant) for all preschoolers in their trial from pre- to posttreatment and at the follow-up assessments across 3 years. Of the 2 studies to recommend increases in outdoor play, only Taveras and colleagues[23] reported outcome data, finding small increases irrespective of group assignment. Only one study evaluated the relationship between activity changes and preschooler weight outcomes and found MVPA was not a significant predictor of BMIz change.[71] Specific strategies targeting PA changes included self-monitoring,[16,18,20,21] pedometers,[16,18,20] working with families to modify the home environment to support PA,[16,20] structured PA sessions,[18] and inclusion of child-[21] or family-based activity during in-person intervention sessions.[16,20] No outcome data were reported on use of these strategies.

Sedentary activity Preschoolers are estimated to spend 52% to 70% of their waking hours engaged in sedentary activity.[74,82] Although many developmentally appropriate activities for this age group are sedentary in nature (eg, coloring, playing with blocks), preschoolers also regularly engage in screen activities like watching television, using computers, and playing video games.[83] Exceeding 2 hours of television daily nearly triples the risk of becoming overweight in preschoolers[84] and having a television present in the bedroom increases weekly viewing time[85] and obesity risk.[79,86] Despite short- and long-term associations of preschooler screen use to obesity,[84,87] caregivers report difficulty modifying this lifestyle behavior because children enjoy it, screens are a good "babysitter," and screens are a go-to activity during inclement weather.[62,88,89]

Although reducing sedentary activity was included as a component in 5 preschool obesity interventions,[16,20,21,23,24] outcome data are only available for 2 studies.[23,71] Kuhl and colleagues[71] report screen use for families randomized to their clinic and home-based intervention only. Although significant reductions in television use from pre- to posttreatment were observed, this change was not a significant predictor of BMIz decreases.[71] Taveras and colleagues[23] found significantly greater reductions in screen use for preschoolers in the intervention compared with the control condition but no group differences on removal of televisions from preschoolers' bedrooms. Screen use reductions achieved by intervention preschoolers did not meet recommendations in either study. In contrast to diet and PA, preschool obesity interventions encourage generalization of a broader set of child behavior management (eg, ignoring, time out)[16,18,20,21] and behavior change skills (eg, self-monitoring, stimulus control)[16,20,21,23,24] to reduce preschooler screen use. Taveras and colleagues[23] also offered television allowance units. No outcome data were reported on use of these strategies.

Sleep Preschoolers currently sleep an average of 11.5 to 12 hours per day,[90] which is within the recommended 10 to 13 hours.[91] However, sleep duration is variable (9.1–14.2 hours)[90] and concerning given its association with concurrent and later obesity.[92] Some research suggests that compared with older age groups, the risk for subsequent overweight and obesity may be particularly high among young children with inadequate sleep. Preschoolers who get less than 10 hours of sleep have 1.5[93] to greater than 5 times[94] the odds of subsequent overweight and obesity compared with preschoolers who sleep ≥11 hours,[95] with evidence of this risk tracking into adulthood.[96] Although the risks for obesity are multifactorial, inadequate sleep may be a particularly strong predictor. Short sleep (≤8 hours) was found to be the strongest of 22 identified risk factors for preschool obesity[97]; whereas adequate sleep (≥10 hours) was the only significant predictor of decreased obesity risk in a model including 3 additional protective factors for obesity (frequent family meals, ≤2 hours screen use daily, and no television in the bedroom).[98] In a longitudinal cohort study of preschoolers, a dose-response association between sleep and weight was reported: each additional hour of sleep at ages 3 to 5 years (average of 11 hours) was associated with nearly a half unit reduction in BMI and reduced risk of being overweight at age 7 years.[99] Similarly, Clifford and colleagues[100] found in a sample of preschoolers with obesity, each hour of nighttime sleep (mean of 10 hours) was associated with a reduction in BMIz of 0.14 units.

Barriers to adequate sleep are more frequently reported for preschoolers with obesity.[101,102] One of the most common barriers noted is lack of a consistent bedtime routine.[103] The predictability of routines allows children to transition between activities more easily[104] and decreases the likelihood of other sleep-related problems that lead to insufficient sleep.[103] Preschoolers with obesity are more likely to have bedtimes later than 9 PM,[102] which is associated with 48 minutes less nighttime sleep.[105] Although the body of research linking sleep to obesity risk is rapidly growing, sleep is not included as a component of any published preschool obesity interventions.

In summary, all preschool obesity interventions evaluated within the context of published randomized, controlled trials to date are multicomponent, which reflects the multiple behavioral risk factors for obesity in early childhood. Although diet, PA, and sedentary activity are included as components in most interventions, sleep has not been included in any interventions despite consistent and compelling evidence for its association with obesity in preschoolers. Understanding which combination of diet and activity behaviors is most salient to preschool obesity reduction is complicated because of variability in the specific diet and activity behaviors targeted and what recommendations were provided to families. Further, most weight control trials do not include outcome data for lifestyle behaviors targeted within the interventions and only one study evaluating the differential impact of lifestyle behavior changes on preschooler weight outcomes.[71] Decreasing caloric intake seems to be the most consistently addressed and achieved behavioral recommendation. Across studies, changes to preschooler PA were low and not significantly different from preschoolers in control conditions despite intervention preschoolers experiencing significantly greater obesity reductions. Findings in 3 studies[16,18,20] that preschoolers were already meeting PA recommendations at baseline also calls into question whether recommendations are sufficient to yield obesity reductions. Reductions in screen use did not equate to recommendations, and few families removed televisions from preschooler bedrooms, which may reflect the significant challenge to making these changes for young children.

Future directions to optimize preschool obesity interventions

Although the literature suggests multicomponent interventions are a promising approach to preschool obesity reduction,[15] research is needed to identify which behavioral components should be included in multicomponent programs, the degree of change targeted, and the most effective and efficient approaches for achieving recommended lifestyle changes and subsequently preschool weight control. The Multiphase Optimization Strategy Trial (MOST)[106–109] and Sequential Multiple Assignment Randomized Trial (SMART)[109–111] are 2 innovative approaches with distinct advantages for advancing the preschool obesity treatment literature in this way (**Box 1**). Currently, no published studies have applied MOST or SMART to develop preschool obesity interventions. However, Brophy-Herb and colleagues[112] are applying MOST to examine individual and interactive effectiveness of 6 different strategies (meal delivery, ingredient delivery, community kitchen, healthy eating classes, cooking demonstrations, provision of cookware) on increasing frequency of family meals and the quality of foods served at those meals. Outcomes will be used to develop an obesity prevention program for preschoolers participating in Head Start (**Box 2**).

Determining Intervention Effectiveness

Understanding what defines clinically significant improvements in obesity reduction is a third important step for gauging progress of the preschool obesity treatment literature. In adult studies, a loss of at least 5% of excess body weight is associated with clinically meaningful improvements in long-term health outcomes, with even greater health benefits after a loss of 10% to 15% of body weight.[113] Currently, no guidelines exist for determining clinically meaningful change when intervening on obesity in preschool-aged children.[15] In this section, we synthesize available data on markers of intervention effectiveness and provide recommendations for future research directions to move toward defining clinically meaningful change in preschool-aged children.

Box 1
Overview of the MOST and SMART

MOST[106–109]

What it is
- A framework for developing optimized interventions or interventions that include only the most effective components and combinations of components
- Emphasizes *resource management principle*: strategic use of resources to gain the most knowledge in a reliable and efficient manner. Design experiments by prioritizing what information is most important for moving science forward.
- Emphasizes *continuous optimization principle*: next round of experimentation begins when the previous is completed; the goal is for each successful round to be a better product.
- Three phases
  - Conceptualization
  - Optimization
  - Evaluation

Example
Conceptualization phase
- Establish the theoretic model: social cognitive theory of change.[16,20]
- Identify components to test: decreasing caloric intake,[71] increasing sleep duration[92–96] and vigorous activity.[81]
- Conduct pilot/feasibility work: pilot test whether home food environment modification with interventionist is more effective than modifications by caregivers only.
- Identify the optimization criterion: BMIz decrease of 0.50 at 6 months.[118,119]
Optimization phase
- Factorial design to examine each component and whether individual effects are strengthened or dampened when combined
- Refine effective component(s) to discern optimal level and dose by socioeconomic status and racial/ethnic background.
- SMART trials (see below)
Evaluation phase
- Compare the optimized intervention with standard of care

How it's different from traditional intervention development approaches
- Instead of testing a package first and then dismantling, MOST begins by examining the individual and combined effectiveness of components first. A comparative effectiveness trial is not conducted until the optimized intervention including only effective components is developed.
- Through use of factorial designs, researchers can answer questions about what components or combinations are the most effective in 1 study rather than a series of studies that would examine 1 to 2 components with a control.

Advantages
- Factorial designs are the only approaches that allow investigators to obtain information on individual and combined effects.
- Use of factorial designs necessitates fewer participants than if the same questions were answered over the course of multiple randomized, controlled trials.
- Effect sizes for components and combinations of components are obtained at each step of development

SMART[109–111]

What it is
- Implemented to develop staged treatments that adapt in response to specific criteria over time
- Design that has multiple randomizations that are sequenced over time
- Randomizations occur at critical treatment decision points and seek to evaluate 2 or more treatment options at that decision point.
- Type of factorial experiment
- Can be integrated within the MOST framework (during optimization stage, refining step)

Example
- Randomization 1: weekly sessions of motivational interviewing versus behavioral intervention
- Randomization 2: at 1 month
  - Critical decision: weight loss or maintenance at 1 month = responder
  - If response, then randomly assign to relapse prevention or termination
  - If no response, then randomly assign to continue with initial treatment approach or switch to whatever approach was not received first
- Questions that can be answered from this SMART design:
  - What is the best first treatment approach?
  - What is the second-line treatment?
  - Is relapse prevention necessary for maintenance?
  - What baseline (eg, age of preschooler) or stage 1 characteristics (eg, caregiver high or low adherence to monitoring) facilitate second-stage treatment sequence tailoring?

How it's different from traditional approaches to intervention development
- Multiple randomizations within a single trial
- Comparative effectiveness trial is not conducted until optimized intervention sequence is determined (no randomization at this phase)

Advantages
- Efficient approach to answering questions about treatment sequencing
- Fewer participants needed than if each randomization was a separate trial because participants are recycled across randomizations
- Can gather information within the context of the study to help with refining tailoring variables (eg, what is the optimal sequence for families with high vs low motivation for changing preschooler lifestyle behaviors?)
- Increased likelihood of reducing cohort effects

Obesity reduction

Within the preschool obesity treatment literature, the metrics used to assess weight are variable. Standardized BMI score (BMIz or BMI SSBS) is the most common metric, but others include waist circumference,[19,114] percentage of body fat,[18,19] BMI

Box 2
Considerations for developing optimized preschool obesity interventions

Developmental barriers to lifestyle modification in preschoolers
- Neophobia
- Tantrums (preferred foods and activities)
- Desires for autonomy
- Activity in sporadic bursts
- Short attention span
- Sedentary developmentally appropriate activities (eg, playing with blocks)
- Need for supervision
- Challenges to playing/staying occupied independently

Promising components
- Decreasing caloric intake[71]
- Increasing vigorous activity[81]
- Increasing sleep duration[92–96]
- Stimulus control for home food environment[16,20]

Important steps to developing optimized preschool obesity interventions
- Measurement of and reporting outcome data for all components and strategies
- Determination of what rate of lifestyle behaviors is associated with preschool obesity reduction
- Implementation of efficient designs like MOST and SMART

percentile,[16,20] and percentage over BMI.[16,18,20–22,114] Within the 6 trials reporting standardized BMI score,[16–23,114] only 4 achieved significantly greater pre- to post-treatment (16 weeks to 12 months) mean reductions in BMIz for intervention compared with control arms.[16,18,20,22,114] In these trials, mean change in BMIz for intervention preschoolers at posttreatment ranged from -0.37 to -0.50.[16,18,20,22] Outcomes were maintained at follow-up time points 6 months posttreatment for 2 trials[16,20] and 12 and 24 months posttreatment for 1 trial.[22] Additionally, although Kelishadi and colleagues[19] did not find significant between-group differences from pre- to posttreatment, significant between-group differences were observed at 24 months posttreatment. Further, in a prospective study of the association between childhood weight trajectories and adult weight status, De Kroon and colleagues[115] reported a mean reduction in BMI SSBS of -0.36 relative to -0.10 between 2 and 6 years of age to distinguish adults with normal weight from adults with obesity.

Although there continues to be much debate over the best metric for examining change in weight outcomes,[116,117] research with older children (age 6–17 years) who are overweight or obese suggests reductions in BMIz or BMI SSBS of 0.25 to 0.50 are associated with clinically meaningful improvements in biomarkers of cardiovascular disease (CVD) risk at 6 and 9 months posttreatment.[118,119] However, among this same age range, other research has documented improvements in CVD biomarkers with reductions in BMIz of less than 0.10 at 12 months posttreatment.[120] Within this review, the interventions to treat obesity in preschool-age children achieved short-term (-0.37 to -0.50) and long-term (-0.1 to -0.50) reductions in BMIz and BMI SSBS consistent with parameters of clinically meaningful change for older children and suggest the effects of intervention on obesity reduction in preschool-age children may be greater and more enduring.

Cardiovascular risk reduction In addition to measures of weight, effect on chronic disease risk reduction is a second marker of clinically meaningful change for obesity interventions. Obesity during the preschool years not only increases the risk for the early emergence of precursors to CVD (eg, large waist circumference, indicators of insulin resistance, and elevated glucose, lipids, blood pressure, and markers of inflammation) during the preschool years[121] but also increases the risk for CVD in adulthood.[122] For example, in one of the few studies to examine the long-term implications of CVD factors during the preschool years, Juhola and colleagues[123] found that abnormal levels of CVD risk in children 3 to 9 years old were associated with approximately 2 to more than 4 times the risk of abnormal levels of CVD risk factors 27 years later. Further evidence of persisting risk from childhood into adolescence[124] and adulthood has been documented in prospective studies with older children.[125] Clustering of CVD risk factors as early as age 6 is associated with nearly 5 times the odds for clustering of CVD risk in adolescence.[124] Similarly, clustering of CVD risk factors at 6 to 19 years of age (mean age, 12.9 years) is associated with 6 times the odds for later clustering of risk factors and more than 14 times the odds of CVD in adulthood.[125] Findings that each 10-point change in age- and sex-specific BMI percentile from childhood to adulthood was associated with a 24% change in risk for clustering of CVD risk factors in adulthood illustrate the broader health impact of intervening on obesity early in childhood.[125]

Within the preschool obesity treatment literature, only 2 studies examined the impact of obesity reduction on CVD risk. Bocca and colleagues[18] explored short-term effects (16 weeks; posttreatment) of their interventions on preschooler CVD risk. Although no between-group differences were evident at posttreatment, the treatment group showed significant improvements in low-grade inflammation. When the treatment and control were collapsed, improvement in percentage of body fat was positively correlated with improvements in glucose metabolism and lipid profile. Improvements in percentage of body fat, BMIz, waist circumference z-score, and visceral fat were also each significantly associated with improvements in leptin concentrations. Kelishadi and colleagues[19] found significant improvements at posttreatment (6 months) for lipid (triglycerides and high-density lipoprotein cholesterol) and glucose metabolism values [insulin and homeostasis model assessment of insulin resistance (HOMA-R)] across the 3 arms in their trial, but these changes were not maintained at the 6- to 24-month follow-up assessments. For the dairy treatment group only, CVD risk factor values continued to show improvement over baseline values until the 12-month follow-up for triglycerides, insulin, and HOMA-R values and significant improvement until the 24-month follow-up for high-density lipoprotein cholesterol. There were no significant changes observed in measures of blood pressure, fasting blood glucose, or indicators of inflammation, and associations with measures of weight change were not reported. Prospective research looking at the long-term implications of change in adiposity on CVD risk among preschool-age children with overweight and obesity is largely lacking from the current body of research and warrants future investigation.

In addition to the positive effects of weight reduction on CVD risk, evidence suggests that change in the health behaviors linked to obesity in preschoolers may have important implications on long-term weight management and clinically meaningful improvements in CVD risk. For instance, in a 3-year, cluster randomized, controlled trial targeting diet and CVD risk for preschoolers in Head Start,[126–128] treatment had no effect on child weight but preschoolers at intervention sites experienced significantly greater improvements in diet (total caloric intake, calories from saturated fat, and grams of fat) and CVD risk compared with children at control sites 1 year after the start of treatment.[127] Among children in the treatment group, reductions in CVD risk at year 1 were also associated with significant reductions in BMI at the 1-year posttreatment follow-up.[129] These findings suggest that although reduction in caloric intake may be particularly important for weight reductions in the short term,[71] changes in nutritional content may also be important for short- and long-term health outcomes.

Although interventions included in this review did not have significant effects on PA, research with school-aged children who participated in an intervention to increase PA compared with children in the control group at 5 and 10 years, suggesting PA may have important implications on long-term weight management.[130] In a separate study, school-age children were followed up for 7 years, and those with the lowest initial fitness levels (lower maximal oxygen consumption peak) experienced greater clustering of CVD risk factors 7 years later relative to children who were more fit.[124]

The literature to date suggests that intensive, multicomponent behavioral lifestyle interventions are the most efficacious approach to reducing the number of overweight and obese preschool-age children.[60] The magnitude of treatment effects on measures of excess weight in preschoolers may also have important implications for reducing short- and long-term CVD risk, which has the potential to reduce the extraordinary annual economic costs (approximately $300 billion) resulting from obesity and obesity-related illness.[131]

Similar to the larger body of preschool obesity treatment literature, research examining associations between change in specific health behaviors and improvements in preschooler obesity are limited, and investigations of treatment effects on changes in CVD risk factors are currently lacking. Therefore, research is not only needed to better understand the short- and long-term implications of specific health behaviors changes on obesity and associated comorbidities, research is also needed to determine the amount and duration of changes needed to achieve clinically meaningful change.

Future directions to increase understanding of intervention effectiveness
Although clinically meaningful change for BMIz has been identified in older children,[118–120] this threshold has not been identified for preschool children. Additional research is needed to determine the most important metric(s) for identifying clinically meaningful change specific to children between the ages of 2 and 5 years. While studies measuring biological outcomes may help to clarify the impact of changes in weight and health behaviors on short- and long-term CVD and metabolic functioning, Bugge and colleagues[124] reported lower retention of participants for data points involving more invasive procedures including maximal oxygen consumption peak analysis and biological measures. However, the combined use of BMI and waist circumference may provide an acceptable alternative to measuring and tracking obesity-related health risks,[121] as research has also found that BMI and waist circumference in 3- to 6-year-olds predicted the same CVD risk factors in this young age group.

SUMMARY

Despite recent declines, excess weight gain during the preschool years is prevalent and problematic with persistent disparities among children from low-income and minority backgrounds.[1,2] Although multidisciplinary, intensive behavioral interventions may be a promising approach to preschool obesity reduction,[15] this review finds that preschool weight control trials have had poor reach to families from low-income and minority backgrounds, do not provide sufficient evidence to determine the most effective and efficient treatment components and approaches to treating obesity in early childhood, and lack consensus on how best to discern intervention effectiveness. Addressing these 3 critical gaps is necessary to advance the preschool obesity treatment literature and eliminate early childhood obesity disparities. In addition to exploring alternative recruitment settings that may increase reach to families from low-income and minority backgrounds and identifying strategies for improving accuracy of caregiver perceptions of preschooler weight status, completion of formative work that integrates user-centered design may improve enrollment. Applying innovative designs like MOST[106–109] and SMART[109–111] will allow researchers to efficiently determine the most effective behavioral targets, the most efficient approaches and strategies for yielding behavior change, and whether and how interventions should be modified so they are optimized for families from different sociodemographic backgrounds. Including outcome measures for all behaviors targeted and recommended change strategies targeted is also necessary to build empirically supported treatments. Finally, assessment of changes in risk factors for CVD and other physical and psychosocial health consequences of obesity is important for reaching consensus on a definition of clinically meaningful obesity reduction for preschoolers.

REFERENCES

1. Ogden CL, Carroll MD, Kit BK, et al. Prevalence of childhood and adult obesity in the United States, 2011-2012. JAMA 2014;311(8):806–14.

2. Rossen LM, Schoendorf KC. Measuring health disparities: trends in racial-ethnic and socioeconomic disparities in obesity among 2- to 18-year old youth in the United States, 2001-2010. Ann Epidemiol 2012;22(10):698–704.

3. Kuhl ES, Rausch JR, Varni JW, et al. Impaired health-related quality of life in preschoolers with obesity. J Pediatr Psychol 2012;37(10):1148–56.
4. Brogan K, Danford C, Yeh Y, et al. Cardiovascular disease risk factors are elevated in urban minority children enrolled in head start. Child Obes 2014; 10(3):207–13.
5. Cockrell Skinner A, Perrin EM, Steiner MJ. Healthy for now? A cross-sectional study of the comorbidities in obese preschool children in the United States. Clin Pediatr (Phila) 2010;49(7):648–55.
6. Margulies AS, Floyd RG, Hojnoski RL. Body size stigmatization: an examination of attitudes of african american preschool-age children attending head start. J Pediatr Psychol 2008;33(5):487–96.
7. Freedman DS, Khan LK, Serdula MK, et al. The relation of childhood BMI to adult adiposity: the Bogalusa Heart Study. Pediatrics 2005;115(1):22–7.
8. Guo SS, Wu W, Chumlea WC, et al. Predicting overweight and obesity in adulthood from body mass index values in childhood and adolescence. Am J Clin Nutr 2002;76(3):653–8.
9. Freedman DS, Khan LK, Serdula MK, et al. Racial differences in the tracking of childhood BMI to adulthood. Obes Res 2005;13(5):928–35.
10. Must A, Jacques PF, Dallal GE, et al. Long-term morbidity and mortality of overweight adolescents. A follow-up of the Harvard Growth Study of 1922 to 1935. N Engl J Med 1992;327(19):1350–5.
11. Cunningham SA, Kramer MR, Narayan KM. Incidence of childhood obesity in the United States. N Engl J Med 2014;370(5):403–11.
12. Barkin SL, Gesell SB, Po'e EK, et al. Culturally tailored, family-centered, behavioral obesity intervention for latino-american preschool-aged children. Pediatrics 2012;130(3):445–56.
13. Fitzgibbon ML, Stolley MR, Schiffer L, et al. Two-year follow-up results for Hip-Hop to Health Jr.: a randomized controlled trial for overweight prevention in preschool minority children. J Pediatr 2005;146(5):618–25.
14. Fitzgibbon ML, Stolley MR, Schiffer L, et al. Hip-Hop to Health Jr. for Latino preschool children. Obesity (Silver Spring) 2006;14(9):1616–25.
15. Foster BA, Farragher J, Parker P, et al. Treatment interventions for early childhood obesity: a systematic review. Acad Pediatr 2015;15(4):353–61.
16. Stark LJ, Clifford LM, Towner EK, et al. A pilot randomized controlled trial of a behavioral family-based intervention with and without home visits to decrease obesity in preschoolers. J Pediatr Psychol 2014;39(9):1001–12.
17. Glasgow RE, Vogt TM, Boles SM. Evaluating the public health impact of health promotion interventions: the RE-AIM framework. Am J Public Health 1999;89(9): 1322–7.
18. Bocca G, Corpeleijn E, Stolk RP, et al. Results of a multidisciplinary treatment program in 3-year-old to 5-year-old overweight or obese children: a randomized controlled clinical trial. Arch Pediatr Adolesc Med 2012;166(12):1109–15.
19. Kelishadi R, Zemel MB, Hashemipour M, et al. Can a dairy-rich diet be effective in long-term weight control of young children? J Am Coll Nutr 2009;28(5): 601–10.
20. Stark LJ, Spear S, Boles R, et al. A pilot randomized controlled trial of a clinic and home-based behavioral intervention to decrease obesity in preschoolers. Obesity 2011;19(1):134–41.
21. Quattrin T, Roemmich JN, Paluch R, et al. Efficacy of family-based weight control program for preschool children in primary care. Pediatrics 2012;130(4):660–6.

22. Quattrin T, Roemmich JN, Paluch R, et al. Treatment outcomes of overweight children and parents in the medical home. Pediatrics 2014;134(2):290–7.
23. Taveras EM, Gortmaker SL, Hohman KH, et al. Randomized controlled trial to improve primary care to prevent and manage childhood obesity: the High Five for Kids study. Arch Pediatr Adolesc Med 2011;165(8):714–22.
24. van Grieken A, Veldhuis L, Renders CM, et al. Population-based childhood overweight prevention: outcomes of the 'Be active, eat right' study. PLoS One 2013; 8(5):e65376.
25. Taveras EM, Hohman KH, Price SN, et al. Correlates of participation in a pediatric primary care-based obesity prevention intervention. Obesity (Silver Spring) 2011;19(2):449–52.
26. Duncan DT, Hansen AR, Wang W, et al. Change in misperception of child's body weight among Parents of American Preschool Children. Child Obes 2015;11(4): 384–93.
27. Anderson CB, Hughes SO, Fisher JO, et al. Cross-cultural equivalence of feeding beliefs and practices: the psychometric properties of the child feeding questionnaire among Blacks and Hispanics. Prev Med 2005;41(2):521–31.
28. Jain A, Sherman SN, Chamberlin LA, et al. Why don't low-income mothers worry about their preschoolers being overweight? Pediatrics 2001;107(5):1138–46.
29. Chamberlin LA, Sherman SN, Jain A, et al. The challenge of preventing and treating obesity in low-income, preschool children: perceptions of WIC health care professionals. Arch Pediatr Adolesc Med 2002;156(7):662–8.
30. Patel AI, Madsen KA, Maselli JH, et al. Underdiagnosis of pediatric obesity during outpatient preventive care visits. Acad Pediatr 2010;10(6):405–9.
31. Dilley KJ, Martin LA, Sullivan C, et al, Pediatric Practice Research Group. Identification of overweight status is associated with higher rates of screening for comorbidities of overweight in pediatric primary care practice. Pediatrics 2007; 119(1):e148–55.
32. Perrin EM, Jacobson Vann JC, Benjamin JT, et al. Use of a pediatrician toolkit to address parental perception of children's weight status, nutrition, and activity behaviors. Acad Pediatr 2010;10(4):274–81.
33. Oettinger MD, Finkle JP, Esserman D, et al. Color-coding improves parental understanding of body mass index charting. Acad Pediatr 2009;9(5):330–8.
34. Dawson AM, Brown DA, Cox A, et al. Using motivational interviewing for weight feedback to parents of young children. J Paediatr Child Health 2014;50(6): 461–70.
35. Cloutier MM, Lucuara-Revelo P, Wakefield DB, et al. My weight ruler: a simple and effective tool to enhance parental understanding of child weight status. Prev Med 2013;57(5):550–4.
36. Fieldston ES, Alpern ER, Nadel FM, et al. A qualitative assessment of reasons for nonurgent visits to the emergency department: parent and health professional opinions. Pediatr Emerg Care 2012;28(3):220–5.
37. Hong R, Baumann BM, Boudreaux ED. The emergency department for routine healthcare: race/ethnicity, socioeconomic status, and perceptual factors. J Emerg Med 2007;32(2):149–58.
38. Lynch BA, Finney Rutten LJ, Jacobson RM, et al. Health care utilization by body mass index in a pediatric population. Acad Pediatr 2015;15(6):644–50.
39. Special supplemental nutrition program for women I, and children WIC racial-ethnic group enrollment data 2012. 2015. Available at: http://www.fns.usda.gov/wic/wic-racial-ethnic-group-enrollment-data-2012. Accessed November 6, 2015.

40. Start OoH. Services snapshot national all program (2013-2014). 2015. Available at: http://eclkc.ohs.acf.hhs.gov/hslc/data/psr/2014/NATIONAL_SNAPSHOT_ALL_PROGRAMS.pdf. Accessed December 12, 2015.
41. Towner EK, Jelalian E, Hart CN, et al. Developing a Preschool Obesity Intervention for Families Enrolled in WIC. National Institutes of Health, National Institute for Child Health and Human Development.
42. Jannise H, Ellis D, Brogan Hartlieb K. Parent focused obesity intervention for low-income African American preschoolers. Michigan: National Institutes of Health, National Institute for Diabetes and Digestive and Kidney Diseases.
43. Foster GD, Sundal D, McDermott C, et al. Feasibility and preliminary outcomes of a scalable, community-based treatment of childhood obesity. Pediatrics 2012;130(4):652–9.
44. Yun L, Boles RE, Haemer MA, et al. A randomized, home-based, childhood obesity intervention delivered by patient navigators. BMC Public Health 2015; 15:506.
45. Czajkowski SM, Powell LH, Adler N, et al. From ideas to efficacy: the ORBIT model for developing behavioral treatments for chronic diseases. Health Psychol 2015;34(10):971–82.
46. Kuhl ES, Hart CN, Morrow K, et al. How do we build it so they will come? Developing a preschool obesity intervention for families from low-socioeconomic backgrounds. National Conference on Pediatric Psychology. New Orleans (LA), April 11–13, 2013.
47. Slining MM, Mathias KC, Popkin BM. Trends in food and beverage sources among US children and adolescents: 1989-2010. J Acad Nutr Diet 2013; 113(12):1683–94.
48. U.S. Department of Health and Human Services and U.S. Department of Agriculture. 2015 – 2020 Dietary Guidelines for Americans. 8th Edition. December 2015. Available at: http://health.gov/dietaryguidelines/2015/guidelines/. Accessed January 15, 2016.
49. Reedy J, Krebs-Smith SM. Dietary sources of energy, solid fats, and added sugars among children and adolescents in the United States. J Am Diet Assoc 2010;110(10):1477–84.
50. Guenther PM, Dodd KW, Reedy J, et al. Most Americans eat much less than recommended amounts of fruits and vegetables. J Am Diet Assoc 2006;106(9): 1371–9.
51. Piernas C, Popkin BM. Trends in snacking among U.S. children. Health Aff (Millwood) 2010;29(3):398–404.
52. Birch LL. Dimensions of preschool children's food preferences. J Nutr Educ 1979;11(2):77–80.
53. Phillips BK, Kolasa KK. Vegetable preferences of preschoolers in day care. J Nutr Educ 1980;12(4):192–5.
54. Birch LL, Fisher JO. Development of eating behaviors among children and adolescents. Pediatrics 1998;101(3):539–49.
55. Addessi E, Galloway AT, Visalberghi E, et al. Specific social influences on the acceptance of novel foods in 2-5-year-old children. Appetite 2005;45(3):264–71.
56. Agras WS, Hammer LD, McNicholas F, et al. Risk factors for childhood overweight: a prospective study from birth to 9.5 years. J Pediatr 2004;145(1):20–5.
57. Carruth BR, Ziegler PJ, Gordon A, et al. Prevalence of picky eaters among infants and toddlers and their caregivers' decisions about offering a new food. J Am Diet Assoc 2004;104(1 Suppl 1):s57–64.

58. Sullivan SA, Birch LL. Pass the sugar, pass the salt: experience dictates preference. Dev Psychol 1990;26(4):546–51.
59. Blaine RE, Fisher JO, Taveras EM, et al. Reasons low-income parents offer snacks to children: how feeding rationale influences snack frequency and adherence to dietary recommendations. Nutrients 2015;7(7):5982–99.
60. Fisher JO, Wright G, Herman AN, et al. "Snacks are not food." Low-income, urban mothers' perceptions of feeding snacks to their preschool-aged children. Appetite 2015;84:61–7.
61. Cooke LJ, Chambers LC, Anez EV, et al. Facilitating or undermining? The effect of reward on food acceptance. A narrative review. Appetite 2011;57(2):493–7.
62. Bolling C, Crosby L, Boles R, et al. How pediatricians can improve diet and activity for overweight preschoolers: a qualitative study of parental attitudes. Acad Pediatr 2009;9(3):172–8.
63. Pagnini DL, Wilkenfeld RL, King LA, et al. Mothers of pre-school children talk about childhood overweight and obesity: The Weight Of Opinion Study. J Paediatr Child Health 2007;43(12):806–10.
64. Fisher JO, Birch LL. Restricting access to foods and children's eating. Appetite 1999;32(3):405–19.
65. Ogden J, Reynolds R, Smith A. Expanding the concept of parental control: a role for overt and covert control in children's snacking behaviour? Appetite 2006; 47(1):100–6.
66. Matheson DM, Robinson TN, Varady A, et al. Do Mexican-American mothers' food-related parenting practices influence their children's weight and dietary intake? J Am Diet Assoc 2006;106(11):1861–5.
67. Galloway AT, Fiorito LM, Francis LA, et al. 'Finish your soup': counterproductive effects of pressuring children to eat on intake and affect. Appetite 2006;46(3): 318–23.
68. Carruth BR, Skinner JD. Revisiting the picky eater phenomenon: neophobic behaviors of young children. J Am Coll Nutr 2000;19(6):771–80.
69. Galloway AT, Fiorito L, Lee Y, et al. Parental pressure, dietary patterns, and weight status among girls who are "picky eaters". J Am Diet Assoc 2005; 105(4):541–8.
70. Faith MS, Berkowitz RI, Stallings VA, et al. Parental feeding attitudes and styles and child body mass index: prospective analysis of a gene-environment interaction. Pediatrics 2004;114(4):e429–36.
71. Kuhl ES, Clifford LM, Bandstra NF, et al. Examination of the association between lifestyle behavior changes and weight outcomes in preschoolers receiving treatment for obesity. Health Psychol 2014;33(1):95–8.
72. Bailey RC, Olson J, Pepper SL, et al. The level and tempo of children's physical activities: an observational study. Med Sci Sports Exerc 1995;27(7):1033–41.
73. Pellegrini AD, Smith PK. Physical activity play: the nature and function of a neglected aspect of playing. Child Dev 1998;69(3):577–98.
74. Ruiz RM, Tracy D, Sommer EC, et al. A novel approach to characterize physical activity patterns in preschool-aged children. Obesity (Silver Spring) 2013; 21(11):2197–203.
75. Dwyer GM, Higgs J, Hardy LL, et al. What do parents and preschool staff tell us about young children's physical activity: a qualitative study. Int J Behav Nutr Phys Act 2008;5:66.
76. Hinkley T, Salmon J, Okely AD, et al. Correlates of preschool children's physical activity. Am J Prev Med 2012;43(2):159–67.

77. Corder K, Crespo NC, van Sluijs EM, et al. Parent awareness of young children's physical activity. Prev Med 2012;55(3):201–5.
78. Boles RE, Burdell A, Johnson SL, et al. Home food and activity assessment. Development and validation of an instrument for diverse families of young children. Appetite 2014;80:23–7.
79. Boles RE, Scharf C, Filigno SS, et al. Differences in home food and activity environments between obese and healthy weight families of preschool children. J Nutr Educ Behav 2013;45(3):222–31.
80. Prentice-Dunn H, Prentice-Dunn S. Physical activity, sedentary behavior, and childhood obesity: a review of cross-sectional studies. Psychol Health Med 2012;17(3):255–73.
81. Collings PJ, Brage S, Ridgway CL, et al. Physical activity intensity, sedentary time, and body composition in preschoolers. Am J Clin Nutr 2013;97(5):1020–8.
82. Oliver M, Schofield GM, Kolt GS. Physical activity in preschoolers: understanding prevalence and measurement issues. Sports Med 2007;37(12):1045–70.
83. Vandewater EA, Rideout VJ, Wartella EA, et al. Digital childhood: electronic media and technology use among infants, toddlers, and preschoolers. Pediatrics 2007;119(5):e1006–15.
84. Lumeng JC, Rahnama S, Appugliese D, et al. Television exposure and overweight risk in preschoolers. Arch Pediatr Adolesc Med 2006;160(4):417–22.
85. Robinson JL, Winiewicz DD, Fuerch JH, et al. Relationship between parental estimate and an objective measure of child television watching. Int J Behav Nutr Phys Act 2006;3:43.
86. Dennison BA, Erb TA, Jenkins PL. Television viewing and television in bedroom associated with overweight risk among low-income preschool children. Pediatrics 2002;109(6):1028–35.
87. Viner RM, Cole TJ. Television viewing in early childhood predicts adult body mass index. J Pediatr 2005;147(4):429–35.
88. He M, Irwin JD, Sangster Bouck LM, et al. Screen-viewing behaviors among preschoolers parents' perceptions. Am J Prev Med 2005;29(2):120–5.
89. Taveras EM, Mitchell K, Gortmaker SL. Parental confidence in making overweight-related behavior changes. Pediatrics 2009;124(1):151–8.
90. Galland BC, Taylor BJ, Elder DE, et al. Normal sleep patterns in infants and children: a systematic review of observational studies. Sleep Med Rev 2012;16(3):213–22.
91. Hirshkowitz M, Whiton K, Albert SM, et al. National sleep foundation's sleep time duration recommendations: methodology and results summary. Sleep Health 2015;1(1):40–3.
92. Patel SR, Hu FB. Short sleep duration and weight gain: a systematic review. Obesity (Silver Spring) 2008;16(3):643–53.
93. Magee CA, Caputi P, Iverson DC. Patterns of health behaviours predict obesity in Australian children. J Paediatr Child Health 2013;49(4):291–6.
94. Tatone-Tokuda F, Dubois L, Ramsay T, et al. Sex differences in the association between sleep duration, diet and body mass index: a birth cohort study. J Sleep Res 2012;21(4):448–60.
95. Fatima Y, Doi SA, Mamun AA. Longitudinal impact of sleep on overweight and obesity in children and adolescents: a systematic review and bias-adjusted meta-analysis. Obes Rev 2015;16(2):137–49.
96. Landhuis CE, Poulton R, Welch D, et al. Childhood sleep time and long-term risk for obesity: a 32-year prospective birth cohort study. Pediatrics 2008;122(5):955–60.

97. Dev DA, McBride BA, Fiese BH, et al, Behalf of The Strong Kids Research Team. Risk factors for overweight/obesity in preschool children: an ecological approach. Child Obes 2013;9(5):399–408.

98. Jones BL, Fiese BH, Team SK. Parent routines, child routines, and family demographics associated with obesity in parents and preschool-aged children. Front Psychol 2014;5:374.

99. Carter PJ, Taylor BJ, Williams SM, et al. Longitudinal analysis of sleep in relation to BMI and body fat in children: the FLAME study. BMJ 2011;342:d2712.

100. Clifford LM, Beebe DW, Simon SL, et al. The association between sleep duration and weight in treatment-seeking preschoolers with obesity. Sleep Med 2012; 13(8):1102–5.

101. Anderson SE, Whitaker RC. Household routines and obesity in US preschool-aged children. Pediatrics 2010;125(3):420–8.

102. Snell EK, Adam EK, Duncan GJ. Sleep and the body mass index and overweight status of children and adolescents. Child Dev 2007;78(1):309–23.

103. Mindell JA, Li AM, Sadeh A, et al. Bedtime routines for young children: a dose-dependent association with sleep outcomes. Sleep 2015;38(5):717–22.

104. Meltzer LJ. Clinical management of behavioral insomnia of childhood: treatment of bedtime problems and night wakings in young children. Behav Sleep Med 2010;8(3):172–89.

105. Mindell JA, Meltzer LJ, Carskadon MA, et al. Developmental aspects of sleep hygiene: findings from the 2004 National Sleep Foundation Sleep in America Poll. Sleep Med 2009;10(7):771–9.

106. Collins LM, Baker TB, Mermelstein RJ, et al. The multiphase optimization strategy for engineering effective tobacco use interventions. Ann Behav Med 2011; 41(2):208–26.

107. Collins LM, Kugler KC, Gwadz MV. Optimization of multicomponent behavioral and biobehavioral interventions for the prevention and treatment of HIV/AIDS. AIDS Behav 2015;20(Suppl 1):197–214.

108. Collins LM, Murphy SA, Nair VN, et al. A strategy for optimizing and evaluating behavioral interventions. Ann Behav Med 2005;30(1):65–73.

109. Collins LM, Murphy SA, Strecher V. The multiphase optimization strategy (MOST) and the sequential multiple assignment randomized trial (SMART): new methods for more potent eHealth interventions. Am J Prev Med 2007; 32(5 Suppl):S112–8.

110. Collins LM, Nahum-Shani I, Almirall D. Optimization of behavioral dynamic treatment regimens based on the sequential, multiple assignment, randomized trial (SMART). Clin Trials 2014;11(4):426–34.

111. Lei H, Nahum-Shani I, Lynch K, et al. A "SMART" design for building individualized treatment sequences. Annu Rev Clin Psychol 2012;8:21–48.

112. Effectiveness of differing levels of support for family mealtimes on obesity prevention among head start preschools. Available at: https://clinicaltrials.gov/ct2/show/NCT02487251.

113. Wing RR, Lang W, Wadden TA, et al. Benefits of modest weight loss in improving cardiovascular risk factors in overweight and obese individuals with type 2 diabetes. Diabetes Care 2011;34(7):1481–6.

114. Bocca G, Corpeleijn E, van den Heuvel ER, et al. Three-year follow-up of 3-year-old to 5-year-old children after participation in a multidisciplinary or a usual-care obesity treatment program. Clin Nutr 2014;33(6):1095–100.

115. De Kroon ML, Renders CM, Van Wouwe JP, et al. The terneuzen birth cohort: BMI changes between 2 and 6 years correlate strongest with adult overweight. PLoS One 2010;5(2):e9155.
116. Cole TJ, Faith MS, Pietrobelli A, et al. What is the best measure of adiposity change in growing children: BMI, BMI %, BMI z-score or BMI centile? Eur J Clin Nutr 2005;59(3):419–25.
117. Paluch RA, Epstein LH, Roemmich JN. Comparison of methods to evaluate changes in relative body mass index in pediatric weight control. Am J Hum Biol 2007;19(4):487–94.
118. Ford AL, Hunt LP, Cooper A, et al. What reduction in BMI SSBS is required in obese adolescents to improve body composition and cardiometabolic health? Arch Dis Child 2010;95(4):256–61.
119. Martos R, Valle M, Morales RM, et al. Changes in body mass index are associated with changes in inflammatory and endothelial dysfunction biomarkers in obese prepubertal children after 9 months of body mass index SSB score loss. Metabolism 2009;58(8):1153–60.
120. Kolsgaard ML, Joner G, Brunborg C, et al. Reduction in BMI z-score and improvement in cardiometabolic risk factors in obese children and adolescents. The Oslo Adiposity Intervention Study - a hospital/public health nurse combined treatment. BMC Pediatr 2011;11:47.
121. Messiah SE, Arheart KL, Natale RA, et al. BMI, waist circumference, and selected cardiovascular disease risk factors among preschool-age children. Obesity (Silver Spring) 2012;20(9):1942–9.
122. Graversen L, Sorensen TI, Petersen L, et al. Preschool weight and body mass index in relation to central obesity and metabolic syndrome in adulthood. PLoS One 2014;9(3):e89986.
123. Juhola J, Magnussen CG, Viikari JS, et al. Tracking of serum lipid levels, blood pressure, and body mass index from childhood to adulthood: the Cardiovascular Risk in Young Finns Study. J Pediatr 2011;159(4):584–90.
124. Bugge A, El-Naaman B, McMurray RG, et al. Tracking of clustered cardiovascular disease risk factors from childhood to adolescence. Pediatr Res 2013;73(2):245–9.
125. Morrison JA, Friedman LA, Gray-McGuire C. Metabolic syndrome in childhood predicts adult cardiovascular disease 25 years later: the Princeton Lipid Research Clinics Follow-up Study. Pediatrics 2007;120(2):340–5.
126. Williams CL, Bollella MC, Strobino BA, et al. "Healthy-start": outcome of an intervention to promote a heart healthy diet in preschool children. J Am Coll Nutr 2002;21(1):62–71.
127. Williams CL, Strobino BA, Bollella M, et al. Cardiovascular risk reduction in preschool children: the "Healthy Start" project. J Am Coll Nutr 2004;23(2):117–23.
128. Williams CL, Strobino BA. Childhood diet, overweight, and CVD risk factors: the Healthy Start project. Prev Cardiol 2008;11(1):11–20.
129. Williams HG, Pfeiffer KA, O'Neill JR, et al. Motor skill performance and physical activity in preschool children. Obesity (Silver Spring) 2008;16(6):1421–6.
130. Epstein LH, Valoski A, Wing RR, et al. Ten-year outcomes of behavioral family-based treatment for childhood obesity. Health Psychol 1994;13(5):373–83.
131. Behan DF, Cox SH, Lin Y, et al. Obesity and its relation to mortality and morbidity costs. 2010. Available at: https://www.soa.org/research/research-projects/life-insurance/research-obesity-relation-mortality.aspx. Accessed December 12, 2015.

Development of a Behavioral Sleep Intervention as a Novel Approach for Pediatric Obesity in School-aged Children

CrossMark

Chantelle N. Hart, PhD[a],*, Nicola L. Hawley, PhD[b],
Rena R. Wing, PhD[c]

KEYWORDS

• Obesity • Pediatrics • Sleep • Behavioral intervention

KEY POINTS

- Use of multiple methodological approaches for determining the potential efficacy of a novel approach for pediatric obesity prevention and treatment can provide a strong foundation and rationale for refining approaches and current treatment targets.
- Systematic study of how sleep duration may affect eating and activity pathways suggests that sleep may be an important modifiable risk factor for obesity prevention and treatment.
- Several future directions are warranted, including further refinement of behavioral interventions, and further delineation of the mechanisms through which sleep may affect obesity risk.

INTRODUCTION

Despite being the focus of widespread public health efforts, childhood obesity remains an epidemic worldwide. The most recent US estimates show that 17.7% (95% confidence interval [CI], 14.5–21.4) of children 6 to 11 years old are obese (body mass index for age ≥95th Centers for Disease Control and Prevention [CDC]

Disclosures: None.
[a] Department of Social and Behavioral Sciences, Center for Obesity Research and Education, College of Public Health, Temple University, 3223 North Broad Street, Philadelphia, PA 19140, USA; [b] Department of Chronic Disease Epidemiology, Yale School of Public Health, 60 College Street, New Haven, CT 06520, USA; [c] Department of Psychiatry and Human Behavior, Weight Control and Diabetes Research Center, The Miriam Hospital, Alpert Medical School of Brown University, 196 Richmond Street, Providence, RI 02903, USA
* Corresponding author.
E-mail address: chantelle.hart@temple.edu

percentile), whereas a further 16.5% are overweight and at risk for becoming obese.[1] Given the now well-documented consequences of obesity for childhood health and psychosocial functioning, as well as associated morbidity in adulthood, identifying novel, modifiable behaviors that can be targeted to improve weight control is imperative.

The observation that while obesity levels were increasing, the duration of children's nighttime sleep was decreasing,[2] accompanied by compelling evidence for the potential role of sleep in both intake and expenditure aspects of energy balance,[3–7] suggests that nighttime sleep might be one such modifiable factor. Numerous cross-sectional and prospective observational studies have supported the association between sleep duration and obesity risk in children.[8–10] A recent meta-analysis found that, across 22 prospective observational studies of children aged 6 months to 18 years at baseline, from diverse backgrounds, children with a shorter sleep duration had twice the risk of overweight/obesity (odds ratio [OR], 2.15; 95% CI, 1.64–2.81) compared with their longer-sleeping peers.[10] The association was stronger among younger (OR, 1.88; 95% CI, 1.26–2.81) compared with older children (OR, 1.55; 95% CI, 1.22–1.97).[10]

Several pathways have been suggested that may link short sleep with obesity risk,[11] (Fig. 1). Experimental studies in healthy adults have provided evidence that sleep restriction or deprivation results in several neuroendocrine and inflammatory changes: impaired glucose metabolism, reduced insulin sensitivity, and increased levels of inflammatory mediators such as interleukin-6 and tumor necrosis factor.[12–14] Of particular interest are the changes that occur in hormones related to hunger and appetite; sleep restriction has been shown to reduce levels of leptin, a hunger inhibitor, and increase levels of the hunger hormone ghrelin.[6,7,15–17] Additional pathways proposed, and supported at least in part by adult experimental studies, include poorer food choices among those who are sleep deprived as well as reduced activity levels related to daytime tiredness.[3–7] Pediatric observational studies[18–23] are consistent with adult experimental studies, suggesting that similar pathways may be responsible for associations between short sleep and obesity risk in children as well. However, the pediatric literature remains limited by the observational nature of most of the existing studies.

To build on previous work, our group developed Project SLEEP, a series of studies designed to determine whether changes in children's sleep lead to changes in eating

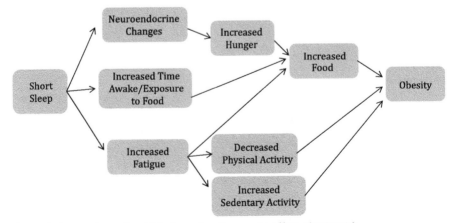

Fig. 1. Pathways through which sleep duration could affect obesity risk.

and activity habits and weight status. The approach was grounded in behavioral theory and informed by empirically supported treatment approaches for pediatric sleep disorders.[24–28] Importantly, studies were designed to systematically build on each other, and to test hypotheses using 2 distinct approaches: (1) an experimental research design, and (2) randomized controlled trials to evaluate relative efficacy of behavioral interventions. The experimental study[29] enabled careful manipulation of children's sleep to create large discrepancies in sleep duration and thus optimize detection of the impact of sleep on eating pathways associated with obesity risk. Given the need for translation of epidemiologic findings for development of a novel approach for prevention and/or treatment of pediatric obesity, randomized controlled trials allowed for piloting of a novel behavioral intervention to enhance sleep. Findings from these studies, the process undertaken to move from one study to the next, and future directions for this work are discussed below.

Commonalities Across Studies

The studies described below were designed with an eye toward dissemination. As such, to enhance ecological validity, all studies were conducted with children sleeping at home and coming into the research center for assessment and intervention visits only. Further, all studies enrolled both children who were normal weight and overweight/obese given that epidemiologic studies have shown that long sleep is protective against subsequent change in weight status in both normal-weight and overweight/obese children.[30,31] Thus inclusion of children drawn from both populations increased the ability to generalize findings for both prevention and treatment of obesity.

In addition, all studies enrolled children who reported sleeping approximately 9.5 h/night (or less). This criterion was used because children in the United States report sleeping approximately 9.5 h/night on average,[32,33] which is less than what has been recommended (ie, 10–11 h/night)[34,35] for children 8 to 11 years old, which is the population of interest in these studies. Thus, as with the decision regarding enrollment by weight status, establishing a criterion for sleep at 9.5 h/night enabled greater ability to generalize findings. Importantly, in the experimental study, enrolling children who slept approximately 9.5 h/night allowed for both sleep extension and restriction by 1.5 h/night without reaching a ceiling for how much sleep children this age could achieve while also not sleep depriving them too much. In terms of the behavioral interventions, enrolling children who slept 9.5 hours or less allowed sufficient room to potentially enhance sleep using behavioral strategies.

In addition, across all studies the authors differentiated between 2 sleep constructs: time in bed (TIB) and the actigraph sleep period. Because children cannot be forced to sleep, but it is possible to prescribe when they should be in bed with the lights out and attempting to sleep, all prescriptions for changes in sleep were made by changing children's TIB (ie, the time between their lights being turned off and the child trying to fall asleep and waking the next morning). However, the primary outcome of interest across all studies was change in the objective assessment of sleep: the actigraph sleep period (ie, the time between when the actigraph estimates sleep onset and offset).

Study 1 Development: Can Sleep Be Enhanced in Otherwise Healthy Children?

Several studies, primarily with preschool children, show that brief behavioral interventions can promote healthier sleep in children diagnosed with behavioral sleep disorders.[25,26,36–39] However, there is limited evidence for the efficacy of behavioral intervention to enhance sleep in otherwise healthy school-aged children who are reported to have insufficient sleep. Thus the goal of study 1 was to determine whether a brief behavioral intervention could enhance sleep in short-sleeping children. Given that it was a first evaluation of the newly designed intervention (described later; **Table 1**) it focused on acute changes in sleep. With an eye toward obesity prevention/treatment, it also focused on whether changes in sleep affected children's eating behaviors. We assessed the relative reinforcing value (RRV) of food, which provided an objective measure of motivation for an energy-dense food reward.

Fourteen children 8 to 11 years old who slept 9.5 h/night or less most nights of the week were enrolled into this 3-week pilot study. Following a 1-week baseline assessment, children were randomized to either increase their TIB by 1.5 h/night or continue

Table 1
Behavioral intervention components employed in studies 1 and 3

Behavioral Strategy	Operationalization
Goal setting	Families are prescribed a 1–1.5 h increase in children's TIB, which is based on family reported TIB achieved at baseline and confirmed with actigraphy
Preplanning	Although the behavioral goal for TIB is prescriptive, interventionists preplan with families how best to achieve the goal given schedules and life circumstances. Flexibility is afforded on weekends (ie, children are allowed to stay up 1 h later as long as they can sleep in the next day for an additional hour)
Self-monitoring	Families are provided with sleep diaries in which they document the time lights are turned off and the child is trying to fall asleep, time the child wakes up, and time the child gets out of bed. Monitoring of mood, aberrations during the day (eg, vacation day from school, illness), and activities included in bedtime routines is also included
Problem solving	Both facilitators and barriers to achieving the behavioral goals are identified. Intervention staff work with families to help them identify strategies for maximizing facilitators and minimizing likelihood of barriers to behavior change
Positive reinforcement	Positive reinforcement is woven throughout the intervention. Intervention staff positively reinforce families throughout intervention sessions, parents are taught to do the same at home throughout the duration of the study, and a sticker chart with family-focused, nonmonetary (or minimally priced) rewards is used to encourage children to make changes in their TIB
Positive routine	To promote sleep onset, families are encouraged to develop a bedtime routine of approximately 20–30 min that includes the use of a routine set of behaviors that can serve as cues for sleep onset (eg, brushing teeth, getting pajamas on, reading a book together)
Sleep hygiene/stimulus control strategies	In addition to positive routines, several stimulus control strategies are reviewed and recommended to enhance the likelihood of adherence to the prescribed changes in TIB. These strategies include a consistent sleep schedule, no caffeine within at least 2 h of bedtime, no screen time as part of the bedtime routine, removing televisions and other light-emitting devices from bedrooms, and using beds only for sleeping (eg, no homework in bed)

with their current sleep habits. The 1.5-hour TIB increase was a prescription designed to maximize children's ability to achieve an increase in the actigraph sleep period of at least 45 min/night (ie, estimating sleep onset latency of 20–25 minutes and not expecting children to have perfect adherence to the prescribed change in TIB). Intervention families were provided with effective behavioral strategies to increase TIB, and returned after 1 week to assess adherence and problem-solve regarding barriers. **Table 1** details the effective behavioral strategies used in this study. A 2:1 (intervention/control) randomization scheme was used to ensure adequate samples to assess intervention efficacy. All children returned again 2 weeks after baseline for the follow-up assessment. Primary variables of interest were change in the actigraph sleep period and change in food reinforcement (ie, how motivated a child was for a food reward). The Behavioral Choice Task,[40] a validated computer-based measure, was used to assess food reinforcement.[41–43] In this pilot, we were specifically interested in the RRV of energy-dense snack foods compared with sedentary activities (that were equally liked).

Twelve (86%) children had complete study data (1 child did not attend the 2-week assessment, and an actigraph malfunctioned in a second child). Children were 9.2 ± 1.1 years old with a mean body mass index (BMI) percentile (using CDC norms) of 71.7 ± 29.3 (58% overweight/obese); 75% were male, and 66% were non-Hispanic white. As shown in **Fig. 2**, children in the intervention condition increased their actigraph sleep period by 40 ± 22 min/night versus a decrease (−16 ± 30 min/night) in control participants (t = 3.77; P = .004; d = 2.30). Children in the intervention tended to decrease the proportion of points earned for a food reward (−0.09 ± 0.21), whereas children in the control group showed no change (0.006 ± 0.04; t = −1.09; nonsignificant; d = 0.56) **(Fig. 3)**. Although this change in the RRV of food was not significant, it represents a medium-sized effect.

In summary, this study showed that our intervention was able to acutely enhance school-aged children's sleep. Importantly, there were no observed or reported negative effects of intervention, such as longer sleep onset latency or greater percentage of time lying awake in bed. Further, there was also a signal that changes in sleep could lead to changes in children's motivation for food. Thus these encouraging results suggested the need to continue to evaluate the potential utility of sleep in enhancing children's weight-related behaviors. However, findings were limited by the focus on acute (2-week) changes in sleep in a small sample of children. Further, it was challenging reviewing with families all of the behavioral strategies (eg, goal setting, stimulus control/sleep hygiene, self-monitoring, and positive reinforcement) in a single visit of 45 to 60 minutes. Thus, to enhance potential efficacy, the intervention needed to be refined to deliver the behavioral content across greater than 1 treatment session. Further, to strengthen rationale it would be important to show that changes in sleep could be

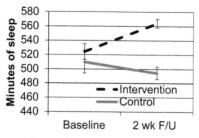

Fig. 2. Mean between-groups change in actigraph sleep period. F/U, follow-up.

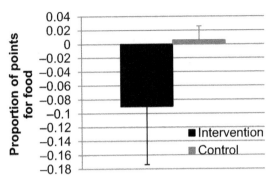

Fig. 3. Mean between-groups change in the RRV of food.

maintained over longer periods of time and with a larger sample of children. In addition, although the primary focus of study 1 was to determine whether sleep could be enhanced in otherwise healthy children, it was not designed to create large changes in sleep to maximize the ability to detect whether changes in sleep affect changes in several potential pathways through which sleep may affect obesity risk.

Study 2 Preliminary Testing: Experimental Changes in Sleep, Eating, and Weight

As study 1 was closing, study 2, which used an experimental design, was being launched. As noted earlier, this second study, a proof-of-concept study, was designed to maximize differences in children's sleep to allow detection of how sleep may affect obesity risk, primarily through eating pathways. Primary findings have been previously reported; readers are referred to the main article for details.[29] In brief, 39 children were enrolled into a 3-week study. During the first week, children were asked to sleep their typical amount. This week served 2 main purposes: to ensure final eligibility for the study based on reported sleep length (confirmed with actigraphy), and to establish a starting point from which to prescribe changes in TIB during the experimental weeks. After the baseline week, children were randomized to either increase or decrease TIB by 1.5 h/night (thus, the goal was to create a 3-hour TIB difference between experimental conditions). All changes in TIB were made by changing bedtimes; wake times remained constant across all study weeks. In order to achieve high levels of participant adherence, several strategies were used, including prescription of bedtimes and wake times (which were closely monitored by study staff through a twice-daily call-in system) as well as children being paid to adhere to the sleep schedule.[29] Primary outcomes of interest were reported dietary intake (measured by 3-day 24-hour dietary recalls), fasting levels of leptin and ghrelin, and food reinforcement.

Thirty-seven of the 39 enrolled children completed the study. Findings showed high levels of adherence to the prescribed sleep schedule with a 141-minute difference in the actigraph sleep period between conditions.[29] Importantly, when children decreased their sleep, they reported consuming 134 kcal/d more (based on 3 days of 24-hour dietary recalls) and weighed approximately 0.22 kg (0.5 lb) more at the end of the decreased week compared with their weight at the end of the increased week.[29] Most of the additional caloric intake was reportedly consumed during the additional hours awake in the evening during the decreased sleep condition. Despite these changes in reported caloric intake and measured weight, there were no differences in food reinforcement or in fasting ghrelin levels. Further, findings regarding leptin were contrary to hypotheses, which may have been caused by several factors, including energy balance not being maintained (ie, children's weight changed) and potential effects of the circadian timing system (given large shifts in bedtimes).[29]

Nonetheless, findings from this experimental study were encouraging. High levels of adherence to the prescribed changes in TIB and objective measures of sleep time allowed a valid comparison of how changes in sleep could affect changes in the study outcomes. Findings also provided a second signal that changes in sleep could affect changes in eating behaviors. Importantly, they also suggested that large changes in sleep could affect children's weight status. However, limitations were observed, including the focus, again, on acute changes in sleep duration and a small study sample as well as a lack of a wash-out period between experimental conditions. To determine clinical significance of preliminary findings, a larger trial that assesses how prescribed changes in TIB affect children's sleep, eating and activity behaviors, and weight status was needed.

Study 3 Efficacy: Does a Brief Behavioral Intervention Lead to Short-term Changes in Sleep, Eating and Activity Behaviors, and Weight Status?

To address limitations of the 2 previous studies, study 3, which is an ongoing, fully powered randomized controlled trial, was launched. Primary aims are to determine whether a brief behavioral intervention to increase sleep in school-aged children results in changes in the actigraph sleep period relative to control over a 2-month interval, and to determine the effect of intervention on eating and activity behaviors, and weight status. Specifically, we hypothesize that children randomized to the optimized sleep condition will show greater increases in the actigraph sleep period at 2 months than children in the control group. Second, children in the optimized sleep group will show a greater decrease in total caloric intake and percentage of their calories consumed as fat relative to controls. Additional secondary hypotheses are that the optimized sleep group will engage in more moderate-vigorous physical activity and less sedentary activity, that they will show a greater decrease in the RRV of food, and that they will show a greater decrease in BMI z-score compared with children in the control group.

One-hundred and four children aged 8 to 11 years who are reported by parents to sleep approximately 9.5 hours or less each night are being enrolled in the 2-month study. After completing a baseline assessment week during which eligibility based on reported TIB is confirmed with actigraphy, children are randomized in a 1:1 fashion to either the active behavioral intervention or a control for contact condition (ie, same number of visits as the intervention arm, but no discussion of enhancing sleep; just a focus on accurate completion of assessments and study procedures). As in study 1, children randomized to the intervention group are being asked to increase TIB by 1.5 h/night over the study period, and children in the control group are being asked to continue with current sleep behaviors. To extend findings from the first 2 studies, assessments are occurring at baseline, 2 weeks, and 2 months. At each assessment, sleep duration is being estimated using standard procedures for wrist-worn actigraphy to establish the actigraph sleep period[44,45]; dietary intake is being assessed with 3 days of 24-hour dietary recalls (using multiple pass methodology), and physical activity is being assessed with hip-worn accelerometry. Height and weight are being assessed by study staff using standard procedures and with children in light clothing and without shoes. In addition, food reinforcement is being assessed as in studies 1 and 2 with the Behavioral Choice task. Importantly, given findings from study 2 suggesting that changes in food intake were observed later in the day, assessments were moved from the morning to the late afternoon/early evening in an effort to capture potential changes in eating behaviors that may result from changes in sleep.

The sleep intervention mirrors the one developed and tested in study 1, but is being delivered across 4 sessions. Given the evidence from the prior studies and the wider sleep literature that a brief behavioral intervention can produce large changes in sleep,[25,26,36–39] 2 in-person intervention sessions are being provided (60 minutes and 30 minutes, respectively) delivered by a trained behavioral interventionist in the first 2 weeks postrandomization: the first immediately following randomization and the second 1 week later. Given findings from behavioral weight control interventions that early success predicts overall success in behavioral programs, this was done intentionally to support rapid changes in TIB. As in study 1, effective behavioral strategies were used to promote changes in TIB (see **Table 1**). In-person sessions are followed by phone follow-ups at 4 and 6 weeks postrandomization. These sessions focus primarily on reinforcing progress toward sleep goals, identifying facilitators and barriers to enhancing TIB, and problem solving to maximize facilitators and minimize risk of continued barriers.

Findings from this ongoing trial will provide important information regarding the efficacy of a brief behavioral intervention to produce sustainable changes in sleep over a 2-month period. By focusing on additional outcomes such as children's eating and activity behaviors and weight status, it will also allow assessment of whether enhancing children's sleep could have important implications for prevention and treatment of pediatric obesity.

SUMMARY/DISCUSSION

In summary, findings from the studies described earlier show that enhancing children's sleep may show promise in assisting with weight regulation. These findings are particularly encouraging given that different methodological approaches have been/are being used and that each study has built systematically on prior work. Although encouraging, several avenues of future study are warranted, including better delineation of the mechanisms through which sleep duration influences weight status, continued refinement of intervention targets, and evaluation of intervention efficacy over longer periods of time. Determination of the relative efficacy of sleep as an adjunct treatment approach for pediatric obesity may also be warranted.

Although several pathways through which sleep may affect obesity risk have been proposed, it will be important to more clearly specify potential mechanisms underlying this relationship. Doing so may not only help to strengthen the rationale for enhancing sleep as a means of affecting children's weight status, it may also help identify ways to further enhance intervention efficacy. For example, findings from our experimental study suggest that the additional hours awake may, at least in part, account for additional caloric intake when children's sleep is restricted.[29] This finding is consistent with other emerging work with adolescents[46] and adults,[3] and may suggest that the increased exposure to food-rich environments is a primary pathway through which short sleep affects obesity risk. As such, interventions focused on stimulus control efforts to minimize less healthy food options and potentially decrease the variety of foods available in the home may be an important adjunct treatment target. Alternatively, given large shifts that were made in children's bedtimes in study 2, the circadian timing system may also be influencing eating behaviors. Emerging work shows a potentially important role of the circadian system in eating behaviors, hormonal release and metabolism, and weight regulation.[47–49] Thus it is possible that shifts in circadian timing could affect study outcomes.

In addition to previously identified mechanisms, other unique mechanisms could account for how changes in sleep affect obesity risk. For example, one mechanism that has been associated with both sleep and obesity risk is executive functions (EF). It is notable that the association between sleep and obesity risk is strongest during a period of rapid growth in EF.[50,51] This observation is underscored by several studies that have shown independent associations between EF and both sleep[52,53] and obesity risk.[54,55] It has been suggested that sleep deprivation may lead to unhealthy eating behaviors and weight gain via changes in EF secondary to functional changes in the prefrontal cortex (PFC), specifically regions involved in reward and regulation of emotion and behavior. Imaging studies with adults support this hypothesis. When presented with food images, participants show, for example, increased activation in the right anterior cingulate cortex[56] and orbitofrontal cortex[57] when sleep is restricted (compared with a rested condition). These regions are involved in motivation, reinforcement, decision making, and self-control.[57] An additional study showed decreased activation to food images in the ventromedial PFC in individuals who reported greater daytime sleepiness (compared with those who were less sleepy), suggesting possible decreases in inhibition related to energy-dense foods when fatigued.[58] Thus insufficient sleep may predispose individuals to excessive caloric intake because the rewarding properties of food (particularly highly palatable foods)[17] strengthen; the ability to inhibit responses to energy-dense foods is impaired; and the ability to sustain goal-directed, healthy eating behaviors is compromised. This hypothesis is consistent with behavioral findings. Experimental studies with adults suggest that increased caloric intake is not caused by greater homeostatic need for energy, but by hedonic processes (ie, greater appetitive drive).[3,59,60] Enhancing sleep could therefore decrease excessive energy intake by decreasing the rewarding properties of food (an effect found in study 1), and enhancing individuals' ability to resist food temptations within the context of our food-rich environment. At present these potential pathways are speculative. It will be important to conduct additional studies to more definitively delineate underlying processes that may be at work.

Beyond the importance of identifying mechanisms, future work could continue to extend the present findings in several ways. Although study 3 is ongoing, if findings are consistent with previous studies, demonstration of persistence of treatment effects over longer periods of time will be important. This finding will be particularly relevant given that enhancing children's sleep for longer periods of time will likely be necessary to observe significant effects on weight-related outcomes. Given the need for translation of empirical findings to community settings, it will also be important to identify active treatment components. As noted earlier, our studies in this area affect both the duration of sleep and parameters that may optimize circadian functioning (ie, advancing bedtimes, promoting consistent sleep schedules). Thus it will be important to determine which component is driving the observed findings (or whether both are key) so that targeted messages can be developed to efficiently promote necessary behavior change. Given that this work has focused singularly on enhancing sleep duration, to maximize impact on weight outcomes, it will also be important to consider combining a brief behavioral sleep intervention with other established approaches and/or strategies for weight regulation (ie, as adjunct to standard behavioral weight control treatment and/or with targeted obesogenic behaviors). Such an approach may be key to understanding the utility of sleep at enhancing weight regulation, and maximizing the efficacy of brief approaches with high translation potential.

In conclusion, our developmental work related to the effect of enhancing sleep on weight-related outcomes suggests that sleep may play an important role in children's weight regulation. Although additional work is needed to more definitively identify sleep as a key behavior to enhance in an effort to decrease pediatric obesity risk, these preliminary studies, along with emerging work with adolescents and adults, provide a strong foundation for continued exploration.

ACKNOWLEDGMENTS

The authors acknowledge all of the collaborators involved in these studies, including Mary Carskadon, PhD; Hollie Raynor, PhD; Elissa Jelalian, PhD; Judith Owens, MD, MPH; Robert Considine, PhD; Joseph Fava, PhD; and Adam Davey, PhD. In addition, we thank the postdoctoral fellows and staff who ensured the success of each study, including Alyssa Cairns, PhD; Elizabeth Kuhl, PhD; Kathrin Osterholt Fedosov, MA; Brittany James; Jessica Lawton; Amanda Samuels; Victoria Mathieu; Zeely Denmat; Isabella Cassell; Risha Kheterpal; Ashley Greer; Heather Polonsky; and Andrew Pool. We are also indebted to all of the participating families in these studies, without whom reporting of these findings would not be possible.

REFERENCES

1. Ogden CL, Carroll MD, Kit BK, et al. Prevalence of childhood and adult obesity in the United States, 2011-2012. JAMA 2014;311(8):806–14.
2. Matricciani L, Olds T, Petkov J. In search of lost sleep: secular trends in the sleep time of school-aged children and adolescents. Sleep Med Rev 2012;16(3): 203–11.
3. Markwald RR, Melanson EL, Smith MR, et al. Impact of insufficient sleep on total daily energy expenditure, food intake, and weight gain. Proceedings of the National Academy of Sciences of the United States of America 2013;110(14): 5695–700.
4. Brondel L, Romer MA, Nougues PM, et al. Acute partial sleep deprivation increases food intake in healthy men. Am J Clin Nutr 2010;91(6):1550–9.
5. St-Onge MP, Roberts AL, Chen J, et al. Short sleep duration increases energy intakes but does not change energy expenditure in normal-weight individuals. Am J Clin Nutr 2011;94(2):410–6.
6. Schmid SM, Hallschmid M, Jauch-Chara K, et al. A single night of sleep deprivation increases ghrelin levels and feelings of hunger in normal-weight healthy men. J Sleep Res 2008;17(3):331–4.
7. Benedict C, Hallschmid M, Lassen A, et al. Acute sleep deprivation reduces energy expenditure in healthy men. Am J Clin Nutr 2011;93(6):1229–36.
8. Cappuccio FP, Taggart FM, Kandala NB, et al. Meta-analysis of short sleep duration and obesity in children and adults. Sleep 2008;31(5):619–26.
9. Hart CN, Cairns A, Jelalian E. Sleep and obesity in children and adolescents. Pediatr Clin North Am 2011;58(3):715–33.
10. Fatima Y, Doi SA, Mamun AA. Longitudinal impact of sleep on overweight and obesity in children and adolescents: a systematic review and bias-adjusted meta-analysis. Obes Rev 2015;16(2):137–49.
11. Patel SR, Hu FB. Short sleep duration and weight gain: a systematic review. Obesity (Silver Spring) 2008;16(3):643–53.
12. Grandner MA, Sands-Lincoln MR, Pak VM, et al. Sleep duration, cardiovascular disease, and proinflammatory biomarkers. Nat Sci Sleep 2013;5:93–107.
13. Nedeltcheva AV, Kessler L, Imperial J, et al. Exposure to recurrent sleep restriction in the setting of high caloric intake and physical inactivity results in increased insulin resistance and reduced glucose tolerance. J Clin Endocrinol Metab 2009; 94(9):3242–50.

14. Morselli LL, Guyon A, Spiegel K. Sleep and metabolic function. Pflügers Arch 2012;463(1):139–60.
15. Mullington JM, Haack M, Toth M, et al. Cardiovascular, inflammatory, and metabolic consequences of sleep deprivation. Prog Cardiovasc Dis 2009;51(4): 294–302.
16. Spiegel K, Leproult R, L'Hermite-Baleriaux M, et al. Leptin levels are dependent on sleep duration: relationships with sympathovagal balance, carbohydrate regulation, cortisol, and thyrotropin. J Clin Endocrinol Metab 2004;89(11):5762–71.
17. Spiegel K, Tasali E, Penev P, et al. Brief communication: sleep curtailment in healthy young men is associated with decreased leptin levels, elevated ghrelin levels, and increased hunger and appetite. Ann Intern Med 2004;141(11): 846–50.
18. Androutsos O, Moschonis G, Mavrogianni C, et al. Identification of lifestyle patterns, including sleep deprivation, associated with insulin resistance in children: the Healthy Growth Study. Eur J Clin Nutr 2014;68(3):344–9.
19. Verhulst SL, Schrauwen N, Haentjens D, et al. Sleep duration and metabolic dysregulation in overweight children and adolescents. Arch Dis Child 2008;93(1): 89–90.
20. Javaheri S, Storfer-Isser A, Rosen CL, et al. Association of short and long sleep durations with insulin sensitivity in adolescents. J Pediatr 2011;158(4):617–23.
21. Matthews KA, Dahl RE, Owens JF, et al. Sleep duration and insulin resistance in healthy black and white adolescents. Sleep 2012;35(10):1353–8.
22. Iglayreger HB, Peterson MD, Liu D, et al. Sleep duration predicts cardiometabolic risk in obese adolescents. J Pediatr 2014;164(5):1085–90.e1.
23. Leproult R, Van Cauter E. Role of sleep and sleep loss in hormonal release and metabolism. Endocr Dev 2010;17:11–21.
24. Burke RV, Kuhn BR, Peterson JL. Brief report: a "storybook" ending to children's bedtime problems–the use of a rewarding social story to reduce bedtime resistance and frequent night waking. J Pediatr Psychol 2004;29(5):389–96.
25. Kuhn BR, Elliott AJ. Treatment efficacy in behavioral pediatric sleep medicine. J Psychosom Res 2003;54(6):587–97.
26. Mindell JA, Kuhn B, Lewin DS, et al. Behavioral treatment of bedtime problems and night wakings in infants and young children. Sleep 2006;29(10):1263–76.
27. Sadeh A. Cognitive-behavioral treatment for childhood sleep disorders. Clin Psychol Rev 2005;25(5):612–28.
28. Mindell JA. Empirically supported treatments in pediatric psychology: bedtime refusal and night wakings in young children. J Pediatr Psychol 1999;24(6): 465–81.
29. Hart CN, Carskadon MA, Considine RV, et al. Changes in children's sleep duration on food intake, weight, and leptin. Pediatrics 2013;132(6):e1473–80.
30. Agras WS, Hammer LD, McNicholas F, et al. Risk factors for childhood overweight: a prospective study from birth to 9.5 years. J Pediatr 2004;145(1):20–5.
31. Snell EK, Adam EK, Duncan GJ. Sleep and the body mass index and overweight status of children and adolescents. Child Dev 2007;78(1):309–23.
32. Foundation NS. Final report: 2004 Sleep in America poll. 2004. Available at: http://www.sleepfoundation.org/_content//hottopics/2004SleepPollFinalReport.pdf. Accessed March 5, 2006.
33. Spilsbury JC, Storfer-Isser A, Drotar D, et al. Sleep behavior in an urban US sample of school-aged children. Arch Pediatr Adolesc Med 2004;158(10):988–94.
34. Mindell JA, Owens J. A clinical guide to pediatric sleep: diagnosis and management of sleep problems. Philadelphia: Lippincott Williams & Wilkins; 2003.

35. Ferber R. Solve your child's sleep problems: new, revised and expanded edition. New York: Fireside; 1996.

36. Friman PC, Hoff KE, Schnoes C, et al. The bedtime pass: an approach to bedtime crying and leaving the room. Arch Pediatr Adolesc Med 1999;153(10):1027–9.

37. Glaze DG. Childhood insomnia: why Chris can't sleep. Pediatr Clin North Am 2004;51(1):33–50, vi.

38. Owens JA, Palermo TM, Rosen CL. Overview of current management of sleep disturbance in children: II–behavioral interventions. Curr Ther Res 2002;63:B38–52.

39. Stores G. Practitioner review: assessment and treatment of sleep disorders in children and adolescents. J Child Psychol Psychiatry 1996;37(8):907–25.

40. Epstein L. Behavioral choice task: for measuring absolute and relative reinforcing value and habituation of operant behavior [computer program]. Buffalo, New York: State University of New York at Buffalo; 2007.

41. Raynor HA, Epstein LH. The relative-reinforcing value of food under differing levels of food deprivation and restriction. Appetite 2003;40(1):15–24.

42. Epstein LH, Truesdale R, Wojcik A, et al. Effects of deprivation on hedonics and reinforcing value of food. Physiol Behav 2003;78(2):221–7.

43. Saelens BE, Epstein LH. Reinforcing value of food in obese and non-obese women. Appetite 1996;27(1):41–50.

44. Acebo C, LeBourgeois MK. Actigraphy. Respir Care Clin North Am 2006;12(1):23–30, viii.

45. Sadeh A. Assessment of intervention for infant night waking: parental reports and activity-based home monitoring. J Consult Clin Psychol 1994;62(1):63–8.

46. Beebe DW, Zhou A, Rausch J, et al. The impact of early bedtimes on adolescent caloric intake varies by chronotype. J Adolesc Health 2015;57(1):120–2.

47. Reutrakul S, Van Cauter E. Interactions between sleep, circadian function, and glucose metabolism: implications for risk and severity of diabetes. Ann N Y Acad Sci 2014;1311:151–73.

48. Morris CJ, Yang JN, Scheer FA. The impact of the circadian timing system on cardiovascular and metabolic function. Prog Brain Res 2012;199:337–58.

49. Nohara K, Yoo S-H, Chen ZJ. Manipulating the circadian and sleep cycles to protect against metabolic disease. Front Endocrinol 2015;6:35.

50. Best JR, Miller PH. A developmental perspective on executive function. Child Dev 2010;81(6):1641–60.

51. Anderson P. Assessment and development of executive function (EF) during childhood. Child Neuropsychol 2002;8(2):71–82.

52. Randazzo AC, Muehlbach MJ, Schweitzer PK, et al. Cognitive function following acute sleep restriction in children ages 10-14. Sleep 1998;21(8):861–8.

53. Fallone G, Acebo C, Seifer R, et al. Experimental restriction of sleep opportunity in children: effects on teacher ratings. Sleep 2005;28(12):1561–7.

54. Temple JL, Legierski CM, Giacomelli AM, et al. Overweight children find food more reinforcing and consume more energy than do nonoverweight children. Am J Clin Nutr 2008;87(5):1121–7.

55. Bonato DP, Boland FJ. Delay of gratification in obese children. Addict Behav 1983;8(1):71–4.

56. Benedict C, Brooks SJ, O'Daly OG, et al. Acute sleep deprivation enhances the brain's response to hedonic food stimuli: an fMRI study. J Clin Endocrinol Metab 2012;97(3):E443–7.

57. St-Onge MP, McReynolds A, Trivedi ZB, et al. Sleep restriction leads to increased activation of brain regions sensitive to food stimuli. Am J Clin Nutr 2012;95(4): 818–24.
58. Killgore WD, Schwab ZJ, Weber M, et al. Daytime sleepiness affects prefrontal regulation of food intake. Neuroimage 2013;71:216–23.
59. Chaput JP. Sleep patterns, diet quality and energy balance. Physiol Behav 2014; 134:86–91.
60. Chaput JP. Is sleeping more and working less a new way to control our appetite? Eur J Clin Nutr 2010;64(9):1032–3.

Effective Patient–Provider Communication in Pediatric Obesity

April Idalski Carcone, PhD[a],*, Angela J. Jacques-Tiura, PhD[b],
Kathryn E. Brogan Hartlieb, PhD, RD[c], Terrance Albrecht, PhD[d],
Tim Martin, PhD[e]

KEYWORDS

- Patient–provider communication • Motivational interviewing • Adolescents • Obesity

KEY POINTS

- Patient–provider communication is a key clinical skill linked to better patient satisfaction and improved outcomes for both patients and providers.
- Motivational interviewing (MI) is a patient-centered, yet directive method of communication suitable for most clinical encounters.
- Emphasizing behavior change autonomy is important, particularly for adolescents actively engaged in becoming independent and seeking out opportunities to make their own life choices.
- Providers integrating MI into practice are encouraged to ask open-ended questions and reflect patients' own change talk back.

INTRODUCTION

The primary treatment strategy health care providers use when treating patients is communication. Providers engage their patients in conversations to understand their medical history and illness experiences, and to formulate treatment recommendations. These conversations fulfill task-oriented (eg, exchanging information, facilitating

This research was funded by NHLBI (1U01HL097889-01 Naar-King & Jen, PIs), the Karmanos Cancer Institute Behavioral and Field Research Core (P30CAP30CA022453-23 Bepler, PI), and NIDDK (R21DK100760 Idalski Carcone, PI).
[a] Department of Family Medicine and Public Health Sciences, Wayne State University School of Medicine, 6135 Woodward, iBio #1120, Detroit, MI 48202, USA; [b] Department of Family Medicine and Public Health Sciences, Wayne State University School of Medicine, 6135 Woodward, iBio #2120, Detroit, MI 48202, USA; [c] Department of Dietetics and Nutrition, Robert Stempel College of Public Health & Social Work, Florida International University, 11200 Southwest 8th Street, AHC5 323, Miami, FL 33199, USA; [d] Department of Oncology, Wayne State University-Karmanos Cancer Institute, 4100 John R, Mailcode MM03CB, Detroit, MI 48201, USA; [e] Department of Psychology, Kennesaw State University, Social Sciences (SO 402), Room 4011A, Kennesaw, GA 30144, USA
* Corresponding author.
E-mail address: acarcone@med.wayne.edu

patient comprehension of medical information, engaging in informed and collaborative decision making, enabling patient self-management) and socioemotional functions (eg, fostering an interpersonal, healing relationship, responding to and regulating patients' emotions, and managing uncertainty).[1–3]

Benefits of Patient–Provider Communication

The benefits of effective patient–provider communication and its relationship to medical care outcomes have long been highlighted in the chronic illness literature.[2,4–10] Better patient–provider communication is linked to patient satisfaction with medical care and medical care providers.[3,11] Patient satisfaction is critical because it is an indicator of how well the provider is meeting patients' health care needs, expectations, and preferences.[3] Multiple research studies have positively linked patient–provider communication to patient adherence to treatment recommendations and better medical outcomes.[5,12–19] Actively involving patients in their medical care affects adherence to treatment recommendations directly and through improved comprehension, understanding, and negotiation of treatment recommendations.[20]

Effective patient–provider communication not only leads to a better medical care experience and improved outcomes for patients, but benefits also extend to providers and society. Improvement in provider communication skills is associated with greater satisfaction with patient interactions,[21] increased self-confidence for treating "difficult" patients,[22] and decreased malpractice claims.[23] Improved patient–provider communication may also pose benefits society as a whole through decreased health care costs.[24]

Patient–Provider Communication in Pediatrics

Patient–provider communication in the pediatric health care setting differs dramatically from adult patient–provider communication in that the patient is a child and the responsible party is the child's caregiver. This presents a dilemma for the provider; with whom should the provider communicate, the caregiver or patient? Research suggests that providers spend more time communicating with caregivers than with their pediatric patients. Specifically, pediatric patients, regardless of age, are typically engaged in less than 20% of the communication in a typical medical care visit.[25,26] When pediatric patients are engaged in the conversation, they are generally included in social aspects and the provision of medical history with the treatment decision making typically completed by the provider and caregiver.[27,28] When providers attempt to increase pediatric patients' participation, caregivers often disrupt this effort by interrupting and responding to questions and statements directed to the patient rather than supporting and encouraging the patient's active involvement.[27,29] This dynamic may have unintended consequences. Pediatric patients, particularly adolescents, report feeling marginalized when they are excluded from conversations about their own health,[30] which may lead to disengagement and disinterest in their own health care.

Direct communication with pediatric patients, on the other hand, builds trust and rapport,[31,32] helps to socialize children into the patient role,[29,33] and, in the adult literature, has been identified as a primary mechanism for patient adherence to behavioral recommendations.[12,17] With the top 4 causes of early mortality—namely, cardiovascular disease, cancer, respiratory disease, and stroke—tied to modifiable behaviors such as poor diet and lack of physical activity,[34] there is a critical need for providers to communicate with their patients to change their behavior in these areas. Pediatricians, in particular, play a critical role in identifying children who are at risk for obesity and these life-threatening diseases and to encourage these children and their families to change their unhealthy dietary and activity patterns early, before the detrimental effects of unhealthy behavior patterns begin to unfold.[35]

The Skill of Communicating Well

The National Academy of Medicine (formerly the Institute of Medicine) recognizes patient–provider communication as a key clinical skill[36] as does the international medical community,[37,38] medical schools,[39–41] and professional medical organizations.[42,43] Although these organizations offer recommendations regarding the qualities of effective patient–provider communication, few offer concrete guidelines for how to effectively communicate. This poses a dilemma for the provider because patient–provider communication skills are not innate. Like any other skill, effective patient–provider communication must be systematically learned and repeatedly practiced.[44–46]

Motivational Interviewing, a Framework for Patient–Provider Communication

Motivational interviewing (MI) is an empirically supported approach to patient–provider communication that is characterized as "a therapeutic conversation that employs a guiding style of communication geared toward enhancing behavior change and improving health status."[47(p2)] The goal of MI is to increase patients' intrinsic motivation and self-efficacy for engaging in health-promoting behaviors.[48] Intrinsic motivation, engaging in an activity for reasons of personal interest or satisfaction rather than external consequences, has been linked to positive outcomes across multiple domains.[49] MI was originally developed to treat adults in substance abuse treatment[50,51]; thus, there is a strong evidence base for its efficacy in that domain.[52] Since its inception, MI has been adapted for multiple behavior change targets, including health care behaviors such as cancer-related fatigue,[53] medication adherence in treatment of those with human immunodeficiency virus infection,[54–56] diabetes management,[57–59] and weight loss.[60–62] Of particular relevance, physician use of MI has been linked to weight loss among adults[63] and children[64,65] who are overweight or obese and is a recommended approach for pediatric obesity.[66]

MI has a highly specified framework that is both patient centered and directive, making it an ideal approach for health care providers.[47,67] The principles of MI, including providing empathy, collaborating with clients, and supporting client autonomy, are elements of patient-centered care.[1] MI emphasizes patients' decision-making autonomy, which is the tenet of self-determination theory[68,69] and empirically linked to increased adherence to medical recommendations,[70] particularly when treating adolescents.[71] In health care, autonomy-supportive environments are those where providers elicit patient perspectives, provide information and opportunities for choice, and encourage patient responsibility.[72] These characteristics are implicit in MI's core communication skills—informing, asking, and listening.[47] Furthermore, MI is consistent with consensus recommendations for working with clients from different cultures in obesity treatment.[73] Two metaanalyses have indicated that MI was more effective with blacks compared with whites,[50,74] suggesting it may be a relevant framework for patient–provider communication in populations affected by health disparities.

Motivational Interviewing's Causal Mechanisms

MI can be broken down into technical and relational components.[75] The *relational component* of MI refers to the ability of the provider to understand the patient's perspective and to convey that understanding in a positive, empathetic manner. These elements are referred to as the "spirit of MI." Although these components are important for relationship building, they do not fully account for MI's efficacy at evoking behavior change.[52] The *technical component* of MI is the specific communication techniques that providers use during MI sessions to elicit and reinforce patients' motivational statements about changing their behavior, that is, "change talk." Patient change talk statements during clinical encounters consistently predict actual patient behavior change (**Box 1**).[52] In fact, 1 study with substance abusers found that patients' change talk predicted marijuana use 34 months later.[76]

Given the importance of change talk to patient outcomes, a primary focus of current MI research is identifying the specific provider communication behaviors that predict change talk and patient outcomes. Studies of MI provider communication behavior have confirmed that communication techniques consistent with the MI framework (ie, MI-consistent communication [MICO], illustrated in **Table 1**) are associated with increased patient change talk[54,77,78] and improved patient outcomes.[79] However, a methodologic limitation of many studies is the reliance on frequency counts of communication behaviors and correlational analytical techniques which limit causal inference. In other words, just because higher rates of providers use MICO communication techniques is correlated with better patient outcomes does not provide sufficient evidence to prove that MICO leads to outcomes.

Sequential Analysis

Sequential analysis[80,81] is a statistical technique used to analyze the temporal sequence of patient–provider communication and, thereby, generate evidence for the temporal precedence of provider–patient exchanges, which is a step toward establishing causality (**Box 2** for an illustration). Moyers and Martin[82] were the first to use sequential analysis to demonstrate that providers' use of communication techniques consistent with the MI framework (MICO) was more likely to elicit patient change talk than MI-inconsistent communication techniques. Subsequent studies have confirmed the MICO–change talk link[83–85] and spurred researchers to dig deeper to investigate which of the MICO communication techniques, specifically, are responsible for eliciting change talk. To date, 3 studies have identified providers' use of reflections as the critical MICO communication technique, that is, empirically linked reflections to patient change talk.[79,83,86] In one of these studies, other MICO techniques, including asking open-ended questions and an index composed of affirmations, emphasizing the patient's control, reframing, and support actually decreased

---

Box 1
What is "change talk"?

Change talk is patients' own statements about their own desire, ability, reason, and need to change their unhealthy behavior. The following statements are examples of patient change talk related to weight loss:

Desire: I want to lose weight.

Ability: I know how to read a food label.

Reason: I do not want to get diabetes!

Need: I need to be a role model for my child.

Commitment language is a special class of change talk that describes patients' intentions and plans for enacting behavior change. Commitment language is more closely linked to behavior change than change talk.

Next time I go to the grocery store, I will not buy junk food.

Table 1
MICO techniques

MICO Technique	Description	Example
Advise with permission	Offering advice, solutions, suggestions, or courses of action collaboratively (ie, in response to a patient's request, asking permission)	Would it be okay with you if I explained what your healthy weight loss would be?
Affirm	Positive or complimentary statements that express appreciation, confidence, or reinforce the patient's strengths or efforts.	It took a lot of willpower to refuse cake at a birthday party, good for you!
Emphasize control	Statements that directly acknowledge, honor, or emphasize the patient's freedom of choice, autonomy, personal responsibility	This is your treatment and you get to choose how it goes.
Open question	Questions phrased to encourage patients to expand on their perspective, thoughts, emotions, and concerns	How has your weight affected your life?
Reflections	Simple: repeating back patients' own statements Complex: repeating back patients' own statements, but adding to the underlying meaning or emotion	You want to lose weight, but you're not sure how to get started. You're worried you might not lose weight even if you change your eating.
Reframe	Suggesting a different meaning, explanation, or perspective for a situation a patient has described	Asking about your exercise plans might be your mother's way of showing your she's interested and cares about your weight loss goals.
Support	Statements that convey genuine support or understanding	That must have been difficult for you.

Motivational interviewing–consistent communication (MICO) techniques are provider communication strategies specifically designed to elicit patient change talk statements. They embody the underlying spirit of MI to support patients' exploration of behavior change.

the likelihood of eliciting patient change talk.[83] An important consideration of these studies are that 2 of the 3 were conducted with predominantly white adult patients who abuse substances. The third included minority adolescents, but was still within the substance abuse context. Our research group has begun to investigate the relationship between provider communication techniques and patient change talk in pediatric obesity.

Effective Provider Communication with Minority Families in Pediatric Obesity

Our research group recently developed the Minority Youth Sequential Code of Process Exchanges (MY-SCOPE)[87] to study communication in MI sessions with minority adolescents and their caregivers in weight loss sessions. The MY-SCOPE is an adaptation of the SCOPE[88] and MISC,[89] the code schemes used in the previous studies of MI's causal mechanism, specifically for minority adolescents and their caregivers. Adaptations included culturally relevant examples of adolescent and caregiver language, examples of adolescent and caregiver language specific to weight loss target behaviors (ie, healthy nutritional changes, increased physical activity), and

---

Box 2
Sequential analysis

In sequential analysis, the data are organized into a contingency table with the antecedent behavior in rows and the corresponding response behaviors in column. The cells of the table represent the transitions between antecedents and responses for a given time interval (ie, the lag). Each transition has a conditional probability that describes the extent to which the transition is more or less probable than expected by chance.

Responses (t2) → Antecedents (t1) ↓	Adolescent Response Statement 1	Adolescent Response Statement 2
Counselor Communication Behavior 1	Transition probability 11	Transition probability 12
Counselor Communication Behavior 2	Transition probability 21	Transition probability 22

---

codes for provider communication behaviors not described in the MISC or SCOPE, such as eliciting feedback.

We used the MY-SCOPE to code 37 MI weight loss sessions with minority families to identify the provider communication techniques most effective at eliciting change talk.[87,90] Because commitment language is more closely linked to actual behavior change than other types of change talk,[91] we examined change talk and commitment language as 2 separate categories. Our research identified 3 provider communication strategies more likely than other communication techniques to elicit change talk and commitment language among both minority adolescents and their caregivers engaged in weight loss treatment:

1. Statements emphasizing autonomy were more likely to elicit both adolescents' and caregivers' change talk and commitment language.
   If you are not ready to cut out sweets, we can find another area to focus on.
   You made that choice.
   You're the one who knows yourself best. What do you want to focus on?
2. Open-ended questions were more likely to elicit adolescent and caregiver change talk and commitment language when specifically phrased to elicit change talk or commitment language.
   In what ways has your weight been a problem for you?
   What concerns do you have about your health?
   What kinds of activity have you done this week?
3. Counselors' reflections of adolescent commitment language were more likely to elicit commitment language in response. In conversations with caregivers, change talk and commitment language were more likely to occur after the provider reflected a caregiver's previous change talk or commitment language statement.
   You are worried that your weight is going to affect your health.
   You want to be healthier.
   Okay, so one thing you will try is eating a small meal at regular times, versus waiting until you are starving and overeat.

Recommendation: Reflect Patients' Change Talk

Our finding suggesting that providers' use of reflections was a critical communication technique in eliciting patient change talk and commitment language is in sync with the

3 previous studies of communication exchanges among adults who abuse substances.[79,83,86] Reflections are a critical component of MI because they not only convey that the provider is listening to what the patient has to say, but that the provider is making a genuine effort to understand the patient's experiences, feelings, and meaning.[47] MI recommendations suggest that providers spend twice as much time using reflections than asking questions and, when reflecting, to go beyond simply repeating back what patients are saying to increase the complexity of their reflections to summarize their understanding of the patient's experience, which conveys deeper understanding and greater empathy.[47]

Recommendation: Emphasize Patients' Decision-Making Autonomy

Emphasizing the patient and caregiver's autonomy was not only more likely to elicit both change talk and commitment language in our sample, this communication technique was also less likely to elicit sustain talk (statements about why the patient or caregiver should maintain their current behavior, ie, the "status quo"[47]). This finding is supported by self-determination theory,[68] which posits that all individuals have an innate need to experience one's behavior as self-regulated and self-endorsed.[69] Self-determination theory has explained exercise participation among teens[92] and African American adolescents specifically[93] and, recently, it has been suggested that MI is the primary intervention method of self-determination theory.[47] The need for autonomy is particularly relevant among adolescents who are actively engaged in the developmental task of becoming independent.[94] When providers use language that honors the adolescent patient's autonomy, rather than feeling marginalized and excluded from their own health care,[30] their motivation for participation seems to be activated.

Use Caution: Providing Information May Not Always Be Necessary

Although providing information is 1 of the 3 core communication skills (informing, asking, and listening) that MI recommends for the health care setting,[47] our research suggested providers use caution when providing patients with health-related information. Even when providers used patient-centered communication techniques, such as asking permission, using the third person, and offering a menu of options, information provision resulted in decreased adolescent and caregiver change talk, decreased adolescent commitment language, and increased in "other" types adolescent and caregiver speech. It may be that in our weight loss intervention for adolescents with obesity, families already had sufficient knowledge of weight loss and previous experience with attempting to lose weight that providing weight loss information was counterproductive. In fact, in our adolescent analyses, provider information statements were followed by "other" patient statement of which 30% were patient recollections of past behavior.[87] These recollections included rehashing past, failed attempts to lose weight rather than focusing on their present motivation for weight loss. To avoid such counterproductive discussions, we suggest providers carefully elicit and consider the patient's current knowledge and experience before providing information related to changing health behaviors.

FUTURE DIRECTIONS
Patient–Provider Communication in Triadic Encounters

Our research group is currently adapting the MY-SCOPE for triadic communication, that is, encounters in which there are 3 participants: the adolescent patient, his or her caregiver, and the provider. Triadic interactions are characteristic of pediatric health care visits and, therefore, of paramount interest. Our goal is to understand if the provider behaviors that evoke adolescent patient and caregiver change talk and commitment language in triadic MI sessions are similar to those in traditional, dyadic MI sessions. To this end, we have successfully adapted the MY-SCOPE for the triadic encounter (ie, MY-SCOPE3) and coding is underway. To date, our coders have coded 40 triadic MI weight loss sessions with African American adolescents and their primary caregivers. Nine have been cocoded for interrater reliability, which is acceptable (κ = .613).[95] Results from this work are forthcoming.

Accelerating Communication Science with Computer Science

Computational technology has developed rapidly in the past decade with topic and classification models offering an efficient alternative to traditional, resource-intensive, qualitative text analysis. Topic modeling is a data mining technique in which a computer algorithm uses a probabilistic model to identify topics (ie, themes) based on word probability distributions.[96–98] Our research group has been experimenting with these models as an alternative approach to behavior coding, such as the MY-SCOPE. As a preliminary test of these models, we analyzed the patient language in the 37 transcribed audio-recordings from the MY-SCOPE study. In supervised classification modeling, a small, existing coded dataset is used to train a computer algorithm to recognize different behaviors based on the speech patterns patients use. Once trained to an acceptable level of reliability, the trained classifiers are used to label (ie, code) new data.[99] Thus, a subset of the transcripts previously coded with the MY-SCOPE were analyzed with several classification model algorithms (Naïve Bayes,[100] Support Vector Machines,[101] and Conditional Random Fields[102]). All classifiers demonstrated promising results but the Support Vector Machine model performed best, correctly classifying 55.4% of adolescent speaking turns.[103] We are optimistic that with refinement these approaches will offer efficient alternatives to labor intensive traditional qualitative coding and, thereby, accelerate the pace of outcomes-oriented communication research.

SUMMARY

Patient–provider communication, although acknowledged as a key clinical skill and linked to better outcomes for patients, providers, and society as a whole, is not a primarily focus of many medical schools' curricula. MI is a patient-centered, directive communication framework appropriate for the health care setting with an ever growing empirical evidence base. Research on MI's causal mechanisms has previously established patient change talk (motivational statements about behavior change) to be a mediator of behavior change. Current MI research is focused on identifying which provider communication skills are responsible for evoking change talk. MI recommends 3 core communication skills, namely, informing, asking, and listening. A consistent evidence base is emerging for providers' use of reflections (an active listening strategy). Our research provides evidence linking asking to patient change talk but cautions providers to provide information judiciously.

REFERENCES

1. Epstein R, Street RL. Patient-centered communication in cancer care: promoting healing and reducing suffering. Bethesda (MD): National Cancer Institute, US Department of Health and Human Services, National Institutes of Health; 2007.
2. Ong LML, de Haes JCJM, Hoos AM, et al. Doctor-patient communication: a review of the literature. Soc Sci Med 1995;40(7):903–18.

3. Bredart A, Bouleuc C, Dolbeault S. Doctor-patient communication and satisfaction with care in oncology. Curr Opin Oncol 2005;17(4):351–4.
4. Trummer UF, Mueller UO, Nowak P, et al. Does physician-patient communication that aims at empowering patients improve clinical outcome? A case study. Patient Educ Couns 2006;61(2):299.
5. Street RL, Piziak VK, Carpenter WS, et al. Provider-patient communication and metabolic control. Diabetes Care 1993;16(5):714–21.
6. Stewart J. Improving the health care value equation: access, the care experience and resource management. Perm J 2000;4(1):56–61.
7. Kaplan SH, Greenfield S, Ware JE Jr. Assessing the effects of physician-patient interactions on the outcomes of chronic disease. Med Care 1989;27:110–27.
8. Jahng KH, Martin LR, Golin CE, et al. Preferences for medical collaboration: patient-physician congruence and patient outcomes. Patient Educ Couns 2005;57(3):308–14.
9. Henman M, Butow P, Boyle F, et al. Lay constructions of decision-making in cancer. Psychooncology 2002;11(4):295–306.
10. Street RL Jr, Gordon H, Haidet P. Physicians' communication and perceptions of patients: Is it how they look, how they talk, or is it just the doctor? Soc Sci Med 2007;65(3):586–98.
11. Stein T, Frankel RM, Krupat E. Enhancing clinician communication skills in a large healthcare organization: a longitudinal case study. Patient Educ Couns 2005;58(1):4–12.
12. Heisler M, Bouknight RR, Hayward RA, et al. The relative importance of physician communication, participatory decision making, and patient understanding in diabetes self-management. J Gen Intern Med 2002;17(4):243–52.
13. Schillinger D, Piette JD, Grumbach K, et al. Closing the loop: physician communication with diabetic patients who have low health literacy. Arch Intern Med 2003;163(1):83–90.
14. Piette JD, Schillinger D, Potter MB, et al. Dimensions of patient-provider communication and diabetes self-care in an ethnically diverse population. J Gen Intern Med 2003;18(8):624–33.
15. Maddigan SL, Majumdar SR, Johnson JA. Understanding the complex associations between patient-provider relationships, self-care behaviours, and health-related quality of life in type 2 diabetes: a structural equation modeling approach. Qual Life Res 2005;14(6):1489–500.
16. Nagelkerk J, Reick K, Meengs L. Perceived barriers and effective strategies to diabetes self-management. J Adv Nurs 2006;54(2):151–8.
17. Matthews SM, Peden AR, Rowles GD. Patient–provider communication: understanding diabetes management among adult females. Patient Educ Couns 2009;76(1):31–7.
18. Zolnierek KBH, DiMatteo MR. Physician communication and patient adherence to treatment: a meta-analysis. Med Care 2009;47(8):826.
19. Aikens JE, Bingham R, Piette JD. Patient-provider communication and self-care behavior among type 2 diabetes patients. Diabetes Educ 2005;31(5):681–90.
20. Golin CE, DiMatteo MR, Gelberg L. The role of patient participation in the doctor visit: implications for adherence to diabetes care. Diabetes Care 1996;19(10):1153–64.
21. Haskard KB, Williams SL, DiMatteo MR, et al. Physician and patient communication training in primary care: effects on participation and satisfaction. Health Psychol 2008;27(5):513–22.

22. Brown JB, Boles M, Mullooly JP, et al. Effect of clinician communication skills training on patient satisfaction: a randomized, controlled trial. Ann Intern Med 1999;131(11):822–9.

23. Levinson W, Roter DL, Mullooly JP, et al. Physician-patient communication: the relationship with malpractice claims among primary care physicians and surgeons. JAMA 1997;277(7):553–9.

24. Thorne SE, Bultz BD, Baile WF. Is there a cost to poor communication in cancer care?: a critical review of the literature. Psychooncology 2005;14(10):875–84.

25. Meeuwesen L, Kaptein M. Changing interactions in doctor-parent-child communication. Psychol Health 1996;11(6):787–95.

26. Vigilante VA, Hossain J, Wysocki T, et al. Correlates of type and quantity of child communication during pediatric subspecialty encounters. Patient Educ Couns 2015;98(11):1352–9.

27. Tates K, Meeuwesen L. 'Let mum have her say': turntaking in doctor-parent-child communication. Patient Educ Couns 2000;40(2):151–62.

28. van Dulmen AM. Children's contributions to pediatric outpatient encounters. Pediatrics 1998;102(3):563–8.

29. Tates K, Meeuwesen L, Elbers E, et al. 'I've come for his throat': roles and identities in doctor–parent–child communication. Child Care Health Dev 2002;28(1): 109–16.

30. Young B, Dixon-Woods M, Windridge KC, et al. Managing communication with young people who have a potentially life threatening chronic illness: qualitative study of patients and parents. Br Med J 2003;326(7384):305–9.

31. Lewis CC, Pantell RH, Sharp L. Increasing patient knowledge, satisfaction, and involvement: randomized trial of a communication intervention. Pediatrics 1991; 88(2):351–8.

32. Byczkowski TL, Kollar LM, Britto MT. Family experiences with outpatient care: do adolescents and parents have the same perceptions? J Adolesc Health 2010; 47(1):92–8.

33. Nova C, Vegni E, Moja EA. The physician–patient–parent communication: a qualitative perspective on the child's contribution. Patient Educ Couns 2005; 58(3):327–33.

34. Yoon PW, Bastian B, Anderson RN, et al, Centers for Disease Control and Prevention (CDC). Potentially preventable deaths from the five leading causes of death — United States, 2008–2010. MMWR Morb Mortal Wkly Rep 2014; 63(17):369–74.

35. Daniels SR, Hassink SG, Abrams SA, et al. The role of the pediatrician in primary prevention of obesity. Pediatrics 2015;136(1):e275–92.

36. Institute of Medicine. Committee on crossing the quality chasm: adaptation to mental health addictive disorders. Improving the quality of health care for mental and substance-use conditions. Washington, DC: National Academy Press; 2006.

37. Simpson M, Buckman R, Stewart M, et al. Doctor-patient communication: the Toronto consensus statement. BMJ 1991;303(6814):1385–7.

38. Makoul G, Schofield T. Communication teaching and assessment in medical education: an international consensus statement. Patient Educ Couns 1999; 37(2):191–5.

39. Cowan D, Danoff D, Davis A, et al. Consensus statement from the workshop on the teaching and assessment of communication-skills in Canadian medical-schools. Can Med Assoc J 1992;147(8):1149–50.

40. General Medical Council Education Committee. Tomorrow's doctors: recommendations on undergraduate medical education. London: General Medical Council London; 1993.
41. Harden R, Davis M, Friedman Ben-David M. UK recommendations on undergraduate medical education and the Flying Wallendas. Med Teach 2002; 24(1):5–8.
42. American Academy of Orthopaedic Surgeons. Information Statement 1017: Patient-Physician Communication. 2000. Available at: http://www.aaos.org/CustomTemplates/Content.aspx?id=22278&ssopc=1. Accessed October 7, 2015.
43. American College of Obstetricians and Gynecologists Committee on Health Care for Underserved Women. ACOG committee opinion no. 492: effective patient-physician communication. Obstet Gynecol 2011;117(5):1254–7.
44. Drazen JM, Shields HM, Loscalzo J. A division of medical communications in an Academic Medical Center's Department of Medicine. Acad Med 2014;89(12): 1623–9.
45. Henry SG, Holmboe ES, Frankel RM. Evidence-based competencies for improving communication skills in graduate medical education: A review with suggestions for implementation. Med Teach 2013;35(5):395–403.
46. Levinson W, Lesser CS, Epstein RM. Developing physician communication skills for patient-centered care. Health Aff (Millwood) 2010;29(7):1310–8.
47. Douaihy A, Kelly TM, Gold MA. Motivational interviewing: a guide for medical trainees. New York: Oxford University Press; 2015.
48. Miller WR, Rollnick S. Ten things that motivational interviewing is not. Behav Cogn Psychother 2009;37(02):129–40.
49. Vallerand RJ, Ratelle CF. Intrinsic and extrinsic motivation: a hierarchical model. Handbook of Self-determination Research 2002;128:37–63.
50. Burke BL, Arkowitz H, Menchola M. The efficacy of motivational interviewing: a meta-analysis of controlled clinical trials. J Consult Clin Psychol 2003; 71(5):843.
51. Hettema JE, Miller WR, Steele JM. A meta-analysis of motivational interviewing techniques in the treatment of alcohol use disorders. Alcohol Clin Exp Res 2004; 28:74A.
52. Apodaca TR, Longabaugh R. Mechanisms of change in motivational interviewing: a review and preliminary evaluation of the evidence. Addiction 2009;104(5): 705–15.
53. Ream E, Gargaro G, Barsevick A, et al. Management of cancer-related fatigue during chemotherapy through telephone motivational interviewing: modeling and randomized exploratory trial. Patient Educ Couns 2015;98(2):199–206.
54. Thrasher AD, Golin CE, Earp JAL, et al. Motivational interviewing to support antiretroviral therapy adherence: the role of quality counseling. Patient Educ Couns 2006;62(1):64–71.
55. Naar-King S, Outlaw AY, Sarr M, et al. Motivational Enhancement System for Adherence (MESA): pilot randomized trial of a brief computer-delivered prevention intervention for youth initiating antiretroviral treatment. J Pediatr Psychol 2013;38(6):638–48.
56. Outlaw AY, Naar-King S, Tanney M, et al. The initial feasibility of a computer-based motivational intervention for adherence for youth newly recommended to start antiretroviral treatment. AIDS Care 2014;26(1):130–5.
57. Channon S, Smith V, Gregory J. A pilot study of motivational interviewing in adolescents with diabetes. Arch Dis Child 2003;88(8):680–3.

58. Wang Y-C, Stewart SM, Mackenzie M, et al. A randomized controlled trial comparing motivational interviewing in education to structured diabetes education in teens with type 1 diabetes. Diabetes Care 2010;33(8):1741–3.

59. Welch G, Zagarins SE, Feinberg RG, et al. Motivational interviewing delivered by diabetes educators: does it improve blood glucose control among poorly controlled type 2 diabetes patients? Diabetes Res Clin Pract 2011;91(1):54–60.

60. Armstrong M, Mottershead T, Ronksley P, et al. Motivational interviewing to improve weight loss in overweight and/or obese patients: a systematic review and meta-analysis of randomized controlled trials. Obes Rev 2011;12(9): 709–23.

61. Brennan L, Walkley J, Fraser SF, et al. Motivational interviewing and cognitive behaviour therapy in the treatment of adolescent overweight and obesity: study design and methodology. Contemp Clin Trials 2008;29(3):359–75.

62. MacDonell K, Brogan K, Naar-King S, et al. A pilot study of motivational interviewing targeting weight-related behaviors in overweight or obese African American adolescents. J Adolesc Health 2012;50(2):201–3.

63. Pollak KI, Alexander SC, Coffman CJ, et al. Physician communication techniques and weight loss in adults: project CHAT. Am J Prev Med 2010;39(4): 321–8.

64. Schwartz RP, Hamre R, Dietz WH, et al. Office-based motivational interviewing to prevent childhood obesity: a feasibility study. Arch Pediatr Adolesc Med 2007;161(5):495–501.

65. Resnicow K, Taylor R, Baskin M, et al. Results of go girls: a weight control program for overweight African-American adolescent females. Obesity 2005; 13(10):1739–48.

66. Barlow SE, Expert Committee. Expert committee recommendations regarding the prevention, assessment, and treatment of child and adolescent overweight and obesity: summary report. Pediatrics 2007;120(Suppl 4):S164–92.

67. Rollnick S, Miller WR, Butler CC. Motivational interviewing in health care: helping patients change behavior. New York: Guilford Press; 2007.

68. Markland D, Ryan RM, Tobin VJ, et al. Motivational interviewing and self-determination theory. J Soc Clin Psychol 2005;24(6):811–31.

69. Ryan RM, Deci EL. Self-determination theory and the facilitation of intrinsic motivation, social development, and well-being. Am Psychol 2000;55(1):68.

70. Julien E, Senécal C, Guay F. Longitudinal relations among perceived autonomy support from health care practitioners, motivation, coping strategies and dietary compliance in a sample of adults with type 2 diabetes. J Health Psychol 2009; 14(3):457–70.

71. Deci EL, Ryan RM. Intrinsic motivation and self-determination in human behavior. New York: Springer; 1985.

72. Williams GG, Gagné M, Ryan RM, et al. Facilitating autonomous motivation for smoking cessation. Health Psychol 2002;21(1):40.

73. Caprio S, Daniels SR, Drewnowski A, et al. Influence of race, ethnicity, and culture on childhood obesity: implications for prevention and treatment A consensus statement of shaping America's Health and the Obesity Society. Diabetes Care 2008;31(11):2211–21.

74. Hettema J, Steele J, Miller WR. Motivational interviewing. Annu Rev Clin Psychol 2005;1:91–111.

75. Miller WR, Rose GS. Toward a theory of motivational interviewing. Am Psychol 2009;64(6):527.

76. Walker D, Stephens R, Rowland J, et al. The influence of client behavior during motivational interviewing on marijuana treatment outcome. Addict Behav 2011; 36(6):669–73.

77. Catley D, Harris KJ, Mayo MS, et al. Adherence to principles of motivational interviewing and client within-session behavior. Behav Cogn Psychother 2006;34(1):43.

78. Magill M, Gaume J, Apodaca TR, et al. The technical hypothesis of motivational interviewing: a meta-analysis of MI's key causal model. J Consult Clin Psychol 2014;82(6):973–83.

79. McCambridge J, Day M, Thomas BA, et al. Fidelity to motivational interviewing and subsequent cannabis cessation among adolescents. Addict Behav 2011; 36(7):749–54.

80. Bakeman R, Quera V. Observing interaction: an introduction to sequential analysis. 2nd edition. New York: Cambridge University Press; 1997.

81. Bakeman R, Quera V. Sequential analysis and observational methods for the behavioral sciences. New York: Cambridge University Press; 2011.

82. Moyers TB, Martin T. Therapist influence on client language during motivational interviewing sessions. J Subst Abuse Treat 2006;30(3):245–51.

83. Gaume J, Bertholet N, Faouzi M, et al. Counselor motivational interviewing skills and young adult change talk articulation during brief motivational interventions. J Subst Abuse Treat 2010;39(3):272–81.

84. Gaume J, Gmel G, Faouzi M, et al. Counsellor behaviours and patient language during brief motivational interventions: a sequential analysis of speech. Addiction 2008;103(11):1793–800.

85. Glynn LH, Moyers TB. Chasing change talk: the clinician's role in evoking client language about change. J Subst Abuse Treat 2010;39(1):65–70.

86. Glynn L, Houck J, Moyers T, et al. Are change talk and sustain talk "contagious" in groups? Sequential probabilities and safer-sexoutcomes in alcohol-and marijuana-using adolescents. Paper presented at Alcoholism-Clinical and Experimental Research. Bellevue, June 2014.

87. Idalski Carcone A, Naar-King S, Brogan K, et al. Provider communication behaviors that predict motivation to change in African American adolescents with obesity. J Dev Behav Pediatr 2013;34(8):599–608.

88. Martin T, Moyers TB, Houck J, et al. Motivational Interviewing Sequential Code for Observing Process Exchanges (MI-SCOPE) coder's manual. University of New Mexico, Center on Alcoholism, Substance Abuse, and Addictions (CASAA); 2005.

89. Miller WR, Moyers TB, Ernst D, et al. Manual for the Motivational Interviewing Skill Code (MISC). University of New Mexico, Center on Alcoholism, Substance Abuse, and Addictions (CASAA); 2008.

90. Jaques-Tiura A, Naar-King S, Idalski Carcone A, et al. Using sequential analysis to predict motivation to change weight-related behaviors in a sample of African American caregivers of adolescents with obesity. 25th Annual Meeting of the Association for Psychological Science. Washington, DC, May 2013.

91. Amrhein PC, Miller WR, Yahne CE, et al. Client commitment language during motivational interviewing predicts drug use outcomes. J Consult Clin Psychol 2003;71(5):862.

92. Vansteenkiste M, Simons J, Soenens B, et al. How to become a persevering exerciser? Providing a clear, future intrinsic goal in an autonomy-supportive way. J Sport Exerc Psychol 2004;26(2):232–49.

93. Shen B, McCaughtry NA, Martin J, et al. African American Adolescents' exercise intention and behavior: does gender moderate the transcontextual model contributions? Res Q Exerc Sport 2007;78:A72.
94. Spear HJ, Kulbok P. Autonomy and adolescence: a concept analysis. Public Health Nurs 2004;21(2):144–52.
95. Landis JR, Koch GG. The measurement of observer agreement for categorical data. Biometrics 1977;33(1):159–74.
96. Blei DM, Ng AY, Jordan MI. Latent dirichlet allocation. J Mach Learn Res 2003;3: 993–1022.
97. Griffiths T, Steyvers M. Prediction and semantic association. Cambridge (MA): The MIT Press; 2003.
98. Hofmann T. Unsupervised learning by probabilistic latent semantic analysis. Mach Learn 2001;42(1–2):177–96.
99. Chen Y, Rege M, Dong M, et al. Incorporating User Provided Constraints into Document Clustering. Paper presented at Data Mining, 2007. ICDM 2007. Seventh IEEE International Conference on, October 28–31, 2007.
100. McCallum A, Nigam K. A comparison of event models for naive Bayes text classification. Paper presented at: AAAI-98 workshop on learning for text categorization. Madison, July 1998.
101. Cortes C, Vapnik V. Support-vector networks. Machine Learn 1995;20(3): 273–97.
102. Lafferty J, McCallum A, Pereira FC. Conditional random fields: probabilistic models for segmenting and labeling sequence data. San Francisco (CA): Morgan Kaufmann Publishers Inc; 2001.
103. Kotov A, Idalski Carcone A, Dong M, et al. Towards Automatic Coding of Interview Transcripts for Public Health Research. Proceedings of the Big Data Analytic Technology For Bioinformatics and Heath Informatics Workshop (KDD-BHI) in conjunction with ACM SIGKDD Conference on Knowledge Discovery and Data Mining. New York, NY, August 2014.

Advances in Motivational Interviewing for Pediatric Obesity

Results of the Brief Motivational Interviewing to Reduce Body Mass Index Trial and Future Directions

Ken Resnicow, PhD[a],*, Donna Harris, MA[b], Richard Wasserman, MD, MPH[c,d], Robert P. Schwartz, MD[e], Veronica Perez-Rosas, PhD[f], Rada Mihalcea, PhD[f], Linda Snetselaar, PhD, RD, FAND[g]

KEYWORDS

• Motivational interviewing • Pediatric obesity • Primary care

KEY POINTS

• Rates of childhood obesity in the United States remain at historic highs.
• The pediatric primary care (PC) office represents an important yet still underused setting to intervene with families.
• Motivational interviewing (MI) is an evidence-based method to help engage and motivate patients.

Continued

Disclosure Statement: No conflicts.
Funding Sources: Supported by a grant (HL085400) from the US National Institutes of Health National Heart, Lung and Blood Cancer Institute. The Pediatric Research in Office Settings network receives core funding from the US Health Resources and Services Administration (R60MC00107), Maternal and Child Health Bureau and the American Academy of Pediatrics. The funders had no role in the design or conduct of the study; collection, management, analysis, and interpretation of the data; or preparation, review, and approval of the article. The funders had no role in the design or conduct of the student; collection, management, analysis, and interpretation of the data; or preparation, review, and approval of the article.
Clinical Trial Registration: Clinicaltrials.gov; NCT01335308.
[a] Department of Health Behavior & Health Education, School of Public Health, University of Michigan, 109 Observatory Street, Room 3867 SPH I, Ann Arbor, MI 48109-2029, USA; [b] Pediatric Research in Office Settings (PROS), Department of Research, American Academy of Pediatrics, 141 Northwest Point Boulevard, Elk Grove Village, IL 60101, USA; [c] Department of Pediatrics, University of Vermont College of Medicine, Burlington, VT, USA; [d] Pediatric Research in Office Settings, American Academy of Pediatrics, Elk Grove Village, IL, USA; [e] Office of Emeritus Affairs, Wake Forest School of Medicine, Medical Center Boulevard, Winston-Salem, NC 27157, USA; [f] Department of Electrical Engineering and Computer Science, University of Michigan, Ann Arbor, MI 48109-202, USA; [g] Department of Epidemiology, College of Public Health, University of Iowa, Iowa City, IA, USA
* Corresponding author.
E-mail address: Kresnic@umich.edu

Continued

- The Brief Motivational Interviewing to Reduce Body Mass Index (BMI^2) study tested 2 MI interventions of varying intensity compared with a minimal intensity/usual care group. Group 1 (usual care) measured body mass index (BMI) percentile at baseline and at 1-year and 2-year follow-up with routine care by a PC provider (PCP). Group 2 included the same assessments as group 1. In addition, group 2 PCPs received 1.5 days of training in MI and behavior therapy (BT) as well as an MI booster training DVD. Group 2 PCPs were asked to schedule 3 MI sessions with a parent of the index child in year 1 and 1 additional booster visit in year 2, although they were given latitude in appointment scheduling. Group 3 (PCP + registered dietitians [RDs] added MI counseling from trained RDs linked to each practice, who were asked to deliver 6 MI counseling sessions over 2 years.
- The BMI^2 intervention achieved statistically significant and clinically meaningful reductions in BMI percentile between groups 3 and 1.
- Key improvement for future related interventions may include centralized delivery of the RD counseling, supplementing counseling with short message service (SMS) (ie, text messaging), and automated systems to provide clinicians with real-time feedback.

INTRODUCTION

Rates of childhood obesity in the United States remain at historic highs; in particular, class III obesity (BMI >140% of the 95th percentile) seems to be on the rise.[1,2] The medical, economic, and social costs of pediatric obesity are massive and well documented.[3–7] Ameliorating childhood obesity rates in the United States requires concerted intervention at multiple levels, for example, policy, community, schools, and health care settings.[3] The pediatric PC office represents an important yet still underused setting to intervene with families.[8] Pediatric practitioners believe that they should be involved in the detection, prevention, and treatment of childhood overweight/obesity, yet counseling rates remain suboptimal.[9]

One factor contributing to the underuse of the PC setting to prevent and treat pediatric obesity is the lack of effective interventions available to clinicians. Positive intervention effects have been reported in family-based behavioral obesity treatments implemented (often by behavioral rather than medical professionals) outside of PC[10–16]; however, results of most treatment studies in PC[17–21] have not shown significant effects on adiposity in primary analyses (a few found effects for subgroups).[12,17,22–28] A second barrier is that PCPs believe they lack the skills needed to engage and motivate parents and families.[9,29–32] Fully 80% of PCPs report feeling "very frustrated" treating pediatric obesity.[33] Thus, developing and testing interventions for the PC setting that specifically help improve PCPs' motivational and behavior change skills is a high priority.

One evidence-based method to help engage and motivate patients is MI. MI integrates client-centered and goal-oriented styles of counseling that has been used extensively to modify health behaviors in adults, including obesity. MI is recommended for the prevention and treatment of pediatric obesity[34,35]; however, its efficacy in pediatric obesity has been examined in only a few, generally small-scale studies, with mixed results.[17,23,36–41]

Many counseling models rely heavily on directive advice and information exchange. In contrast, in MI, clients themselves do much of the psychological work. An MI counselor generally avoids direct attempts to convince or persuade and is careful not to begin action planning before strong, high-quality motivation is solidified. Clients are encouraged to think about and verbally express their own reasons for and against change and how their current behavior has an impact on their life and family goals and core values. Ambivalence and resistance are explored prior to moving toward action. An effective MI practitioner is able to strategically balance the need to "comfort the afflicted" and "afflict the comfortable"; to balance the expression of empathy with the need to build discrepancy for change; and to disrupt the defenses that have been built around the problem behavior.[42,43]

Whereas the essence of MI lies in its spirit, specific techniques help ensure such spirit is evoked. Two central skills to achieve this are reflective listening and eliciting change talk. *Reflective listening* can be conceptualized as a form of hypothesis testing. The hypothesis can be stated in generic terms, such as, "If I heard you correctly, this is what I think you are saying or why are you saying this..." or "Where you might be going with this." The goals of reflecting include demonstrating empathy and understanding and affirming a client's thoughts and feelings. MI assumes that individuals are more likely to act on that which they voice themselves[44] and they can be guided to help uncover powerful reasons for change through the counseling process. This expression of desire and reasons for change is called *change talk*.[45] Eliciting and reinforcing change talk has emerged as an essential active ingredient of MI.[46–51] Evidence for the causal role of change talk includes the association between the amount and trajectory of client change talk expressed within session and subsequent behavioral outcomes[47,52–55] as well as studies demonstrating that specific therapist behaviors (and training activities) can facilitate its expression.[46,48,49,52,53,56]

Interventions that provide PCPs skills in motivational and behavioral counseling could help fulfill the promise of PC as an important setting to deliver pediatric obesity counseling. This article summarizes the methods, outcomes, and process from the BMI^2 study, a large trial conducted in PC pediatric offices, and concludes with recommendations for improving the intervention and increasing its dissemination.

METHODS

The BMI^2 study (2007–2013) was a cluster-randomized trial among 42 PC practices[18,19] that tested 2 MI interventions of varying intensity compared with a minimal-intensity/usual care group. Clinical practices served as the unit of randomization and analysis. Group 1 (usual care) measured BMI percentile at baseline and at 1-year and 2-year follow-up with routine care by the PCP.[18] Group 1 PCPs received a half-day study orientation and a review of current pediatric obesity guidelines.[35,57] At the end of the study, group 1 PCPs received complete MI training. Group 2 included the same assessments as group 1. In addition, group 2 PCPs received 1.5 days of training in MI and BT as well as an MI booster training DVD. Group 2 PCPs were asked to schedule 3 MI sessions with a parent of the index child in year 1 and 1 additional booster visit in year 2, although they were given latitude in appointment scheduling. To guide their counseling, they were provided with a food and activity screener (described later).[19] Group 3 (PCP + RD) included the same intervention as group 2 but added MI counseling from trained RDs linked to each practice, who were asked to deliver 6 MI counseling sessions over 2 years. RDs were given flexibility with scheduling, although they were encouraged to frontload contacts in year 1. The RD sessions were delivered both in person (required for visit 1) and by phone. RDs received 1.5 days of MI and BT training and the MI DVD.[18,19] They were trained together with their partner PCPs for most of the MI training, although there were a few breakout sessions for RDs only.

Outcomes

The primary outcome was the child's BMI percentile at 2-year follow-up. Secondary outcomes included parent report of the child's screen time, physical activity, intake of fruits and vegetables, and sugar-sweetened beverages. Parental self-reported grades for key obesity-related behaviors were also assessed.

Parent Questionnaire

Parents in all groups completed a questionnaire at baseline and at 1-year and 2-year follow-up. The questionnaire assessed secondary behavioral outcomes and for groups 2 and 3 also provided both the PCPs and RDs with discussion starting points for their behavioral counseling.[18] Intake of sugar-sweetened drinks was assessed by querying, "How many glasses or 12-oz cans of each beverage does your child drink on a typical day?" There were 4 options: fruit drinks, sports drinks, regular soda, and sweet tea. For physical activity, the question asked was, "On a typical weekday/weekend day, how many hours is your child involved in sports or active play?" Screen time was assessed with, "How many hours of TV does your child watch on a typical weekday/weekend day including evenings?" and "How many hours of video games does your child play on a typical weekday/weekend day including evenings?" Weekend and weekday hours were averaged to estimate total screen time per day.[18] Fruit and vegetable intake was assessed with, "How many servings of fruits (excluding juice) does your child eat on a typical day?" and "How many servings of vegetables (excluding potatoes) does your child eat on a typical day?" The 2 items were summed. Most measures used in BMI[2] were adapted from existing instruments. More details about the measures can be found elsewhere.[18]

Parent Grade of Child Behavior

Parents were asked to grade their child on a scale from A (great/healthy) to F (poor/unhealthy) for 8 behaviors: snack foods, sweetened beverages, eating out at restaurants, fruits, vegetables, TV/screen time, video games/computer games, and physical activity/exercise. All responses were coded as "A" or "not A" and used as a secondary outcome, comparing the odds of responding A with all other grades combined.[18]

Demographics

Parents reported annual household income using 8 contiguous categories, which were collapsed into "less than $40,000" and "greater than or equal to $40,000." Education was assessed with 7 categories, which were collapsed into "less than college graduate" and "college graduate or greater." Insurance coverage was queried first by asking if the child had any insurance and then by asking about specific types, for example, private or Medicaid. These variables were used as covariates and potential effect modifiers.

The target population was children ages 2 to 8 years old with a BMI greater than 85th and less than or equal to 97th percentile based on Centers for Disease Control and Prevention cutpoints.[58] Youth above the 97th percentile of BMI were excluded because of concern that at higher levels of BMI, many clinicians would initiate metabolic screening and likely refer the child to a specialist, which would likely differ across practices, introducing a potential confound.

Exclusion criteria were type 1 diabetes mellitus or type 2 diabetes mellitus; non–English speaking parent; no working telephone; child with chronic medical disorders; chromosomal disorders, syndromes, and nonambulatory conditions; medications known to affect growth and mood; and enrollment in a weight-loss program or seen by weight-loss specialist in the past 12 months. Eligibility was initially determined by the study practices and then confirmed by the study team. Those enrolled by practices but subsequently found ineligible by the study team were allowed to continue in the study, but their data were excluded in all analyses.

Study Sites

All practices were recruited from the American Academy of Pediatrics Pediatric Research in Office Settings (PROS) network. Established by the American Academy of Pediatrics in 1986, PROS is the largest pediatric PC research network in the nation, comprising more than 1600 practitioners from more than 700 pediatric practices. PROS practitioners are similar to their broader counterparts, with respect to vision screening,[59] management of child behavior problems,[60] and specialty referrals.[59,61,62]

PROS sites were approached that had previously participated in at least 1 prior research project, excluding (1) sites that offered a structured obesity treatment program and (2) clinicians with extensive experience with MI. Each practice identified an office staff member who served as the local study coordinator and this person attended the protocol training. Practices were asked to enroll at least 20, and up to 25, eligible children. Given the higher rates of overweight and obesity in minority children, oversampled practices were oversampled with at least 25% black and/or Hispanic patients. The goal was to accrue approximately 25% black and 25% Hispanic patients.

Identifying and Recruiting Dietitians

RDs for group 3 were selected from a registry of practicing dietitians within the Dietetics Practice-Based Research Network of the Academy of Nutrition and Dietetics. RDs were paired with a practice. Potential RDs were interviewed to assess their potential for implementing MI using a simulated patient encounter. A total of 15 RDs were recruited and trained in MI.

Motivational Interviewing Training

A mix of didactic and experiential activities was used, following the reveal-practice-reveal model, with real-time constructive feedback. Rather than positioning MI as an entirely new model for PCPs and RDs, MI was integrated into their current counseling culture. For pediatricians, how to integrate MI within the culture of anticipatory guidance was demonstrated, whereas for RDs, integration of MI within traditional nutrition counseling was discussed. The 1.5-day training included the following components:

1. Conceptual overview of MI: its spirit and essential strategies
2. Comparison of MI to other models of counseling and patient education
3. Conceptual application of MI to prevention and treatment of pediatric obesity
4. Integration of MI with anticipatory guidance and nutrition counseling
5. Constructing effective open-ended questions
6. Reflective listening
7. Eliciting change talk using 0 to 10 importance and confidence rulers and values clarification
8. Providing information and advice MI-style (also known as elicit-provide-elicit)
9. Counseling by telephone (for RDs)

Emphasis was placed on eliciting and magnifying change talk from parents, and clinicians were given several techniques to do so. First, they were trained to use the importance/confidence rulers.[45,63–65] This begins with 2 questions: (1) "On a scale from zero to ten, with ten being the highest, how *important* is it for you to have your child [insert behavior of choice]?" and (2) "On a scale from zero to ten with ten being the highest, assuming you wanted to change this behavior, how *confident* are you that they could?"[63–65] Counselors then probed with, "Why did you not choose a lower number?" followed by, "What would it take to get you to a higher number?" A second technique to elicit change talk was the value linkage.[45] For this, parents were given a list of values for themselves and their families, then asked, how, if at all, they might connect their child's physical activity and diet behaviors to their personal and family goals and values.[18,42,43] A key challenge for MI clinicians is determining when and how to transition from building motivation to planning a course of action. To this end, PCPs and RDs were trained in a 3-phase model of MI comprising Explore, Guide, and Choose.[18,42,43,66,67] This 3-phase model is similar to the 4-process model recently proposed by Miller and Rollnick.[51] To help PCPs and RDs experience the benefits of MI, they were asked during practice exercises to use behaviors from their own lives to gain insight about what their patients may experience when they are being counseled. There is considerable evidence that health professionals can effectively implement MI with this type and intensity of training.[68–77]

Assessing Practitioner Fidelity

At the end of the 1.5 day MI training, all PCPs and RDs counseled a standardized patient, typically played by study staff. These encounters were videotaped and rated with a validated MI fidelity scale (available from the first author).[78] Although clinicians were at the training, they received detailed feedback from study staff about their counseling encounter. Practitioners were offered an additional supervision session by telephone. All groups 2 and 3 practitioners who completed the training, regardless of skill level, were allowed to participate in the trial.

Target Behaviors and Intervention Strategies in Groups 2 and 3

Both PCPs and RDs focused their counseling on dietary and activity behaviors shown to affect children's weight[34,79–81] based on Academy of Nutrition and Dietetics and other evidence-based guidelines.[34,82] Snack foods, sugar-sweetened beverages, fruits, vegetables, screen time, and physical activity were targeted. Target behaviors were identified with the brief screener (discussed previously). For each of these targets, parents indicated the frequency of the behavior as well as their family grade (A through F). PCPs were asked to provide positive feedback for green behaviors and then, collaboratively with the parent, to identify red or yellow behaviors that might be addressed during the project. RDs were provided with a copy of the parent baseline questionnaire responses prior to their first session. Group 3 PCPs and RDs were given a form to record their patient encounters which, to promote continuity of care, were shared by providers.

Educational Materials

Group 1 PCPs distributed a set of mostly preexisting educational materials that addressed healthy eating and exercise. All group 1 parents received the same set of materials. For groups 2 and 3, either preexisting materials or new materials that were written in a style consistent with MI and self-determination theory[83] were used. Content emphasized child choice in making behavior change. Groups 2 and 3 also were offered self-monitoring logs for the child and/or parent to complete. For groups 2 and 3, clinicians offered only the educational materials and logs that were either requested by the patient or that related to the target behavior change that was chosen by the family.

Sample Size Calculations

The study was powered to detect a 3-point difference in BMI percentile between any pair of study groups at 2-year follow-up, with an assumed SD for BMI percentile between 4 and 6, power of 0.80, and 2-tailed α of 0.05. Sample size was inflated to account for practice-level clustering,[84] assuming a practice-level intraclass correlation between 0.01 and 0.05. Based on these assumptions and projected 25% to 30% attrition at 2-year follow-up, 10 to 12 practices per arm (30–36 total) and an average of 15 to 20 children per practice at baseline were required.

Outcome Analysis

The primary outcome was BMI percentile at 2-year follow-up. To control for cluster randomization effects, mixed effects regression with children nested within their practice was used. Although the primary analyses are based on intention to treat, post hoc exploratory results stratified by low-dose and high-dose MI received for groups 2 and 3 were provided. Of the expected dose (3 sessions for group 2 and 8 sessions for group 3), 75% was used as the cutoff for low and high MI exposure.

Mean differences in parent-reported child behaviors were used as well as the odds (using logistic regression) of parents assigning their family an A grade for each target behavior. Initial covariates included in all outcome models were child age, gender, and baseline value for the variable of interest as well as all variables that differed between study groups at baseline. Covariates unrelated ($P>.10$) to the outcome were removed from the final model.

RESULTS
Sample Description

Mean baseline BMI percentile was 91.9, with values similar across the 3 experimental groups. Mean age was 5.1, with groups 2 and 3 recruiting older children than group 1. Parent BMI, calculated from self-reported heights and weights, was highest in group 2. The child sample was 57% female and 91% of the responding parents were mothers. Groups 2 and 3 had a greater percentage of mothers as respondents than group 1. With regard to ethnicity/race, the cohort was 60% white, 22% Hispanic, 7% black, and 6% Asian, and the 3 groups differed significantly with regard to ethnic/racial composition. Overall, approximately 68% of parents reported household income at or above $40,000 per year, with group 2 significantly less likely to report greater than $40,000 income. Approximately 39% of the sample reported at least a college education, with group 2 having lower rates than groups 1 and 3. Group 2 was less likely to have private insurance and more likely to have Medicaid coverage (data not shown).

A total of 674 participants were recruited. Data about the number of parents who refused to participate were unable to be collected so the study uptake rate cannot be provided. Of these, 29 were ineligible because their BMI percentile, when verified by study staff, was outside the eligible range. They were allowed to continue in the project but their data were excluded. Of the original 42 practices, one group 1 practice was excluded for not following the protocol; three group 2 practices dropped out (1 PCP passed away, 1 retired, and 1 declined to recruit any patients), and one1 group 3 practice dropped out due to medical illness.

Of the 645 eligible baseline children, 2-year follow-up BMI data were obtained for 457 (71%). The retained cohort was similar to those lost to follow-up with regard to BMI percentile, age, and gender. Those lost to follow-up, however, were significantly more likely to be black or Hispanic, to come from households with less than $40,000 income, and to have lower parental education. They were also more likely to have

Medicaid. Parents lost to follow-up had higher baseline self-reported BMI. The intra-class correlation of year 2 BMI percentile due to practice-level clustering was 0.04 (data not shown).

Motivational Interviewing Dose in Groups 2 and 3

The expected dose from PCPs in groups 2 and 3 was 4 sessions and for group 3, 6 additional sessions from the RDs (10 total). The mean MI doses for PCPs were 3.4 and 3.3 in groups 2 and 3, respectively.[19] For group 2, 83% of PCPs delivered 3 or more sessions whereas in group 3, 75% delivered 3 or more. Thus, PCPs were able to deliver the expected dose of MI counseling. For group 3, however, the mean dose for RD contacts was only 2.7 (of 6). For RDs, only 12% delivered all 6 sessions, with 20% delivering 4 to 5 sessions. Parents were given a choice as to in-person or telephone for conducting contacts 2 to 6, and a majority of these contacts, 79%, were by completed by telephone (**Table 1**).

Body Mass Index Percentile Results

At 2-year follow-up, the adjusted BMI percentile rates were 90.3, 88.1, and 87.1 for group 1, group 2, and group 3 respectively.[19] There was an overall group effect ($P = .049$). Planned contrasts showed that group 3 was significantly ($P = .02$) lower than group 1. The group 2 mean was marginally lower than group 1 ($P = .11$). The net difference in BMI percentile between groups 3 and 1 was 3.2 BMI percentile units and 2.2 percentile units between groups 2 and 1.

Using individual-level difference score in BMI percentile (baseline–year 2), means were 1.8, 3.8, and 4.9 BMI percentile units across groups 1, 2, and 3, respectively, with significance patterns virtually identical to those observed using BMI percentile. The net difference using this method, between groups 3 and 1, was 3.1 BMI percentile units and 2.0 percentile units between groups 2 and 1.

Using raw BMI units, the differences between group 1 and groups 2 and 3 were 0.5 and 0.6 BMI units, respectively (see last column in **Table 2**).

None of the factors- child gender, child age, child race, baseline BMI, parent income, parent education, or parent BMI moderated intervention effects.

Dose-Response Effects

Exploratory completers analyses indicated that across the 5 groups (ie, usual care, low PCP dose, high PCP dose, low PCP + RD dose, and high PCP + RD dose), the mean changes in BMI percentile scores were 1.7, 3.2, 4.2, 4.6, and 5.5. Both group 3 high-dose and low-dose means were significantly greater than group 1. Neither group 2 high-dose nor low-dose means differed from group 1 (**Table 3**).

Table 1
Number and percent of motivational interview sessions completed by the intervention group in the Brief Motivational Interviewing to Reduce Body Mass Index

	Number of Completed Motivational Interview Contacts						
Study Group	0	1	2	3	4	5	6
Group 2 PCPs (n = 145)	3 2.1%	14 9.7%	8 5.5%	14 9.7%	106 73.1%	NA	NA
Group 3 PCPs (n = 154)	3 1.9%	18 11.7%	17 11.0%	12 7.8%	104 67.5%	NA	NA
Group 3 RDs (n = 154)	21 13.6%	24 15.6%	29 18.8%	30 19.5%	22 14.3%	9 5.8%	19 12.3%

Table 2
Year 2 adjusted body mass index percentile,[19] percentile change, and raw body mass index by study group—Brief Motivational Interviewing to Reduce Body Mass Index

Study Group	N	Year 2 Body Mass Index Percentile[a] (SE)	Body Mass Index Percentile Difference[a,b] (SE)	Raw Body Mass Index
Group 1	158	90.3[1] (0.94)	1.8[1] (0.98)	19.75[1] (0.17)
Group 2	145	88.1 (0.94)	3.8 (0.96)	19.33 (0.18)
Group 3	154	87.1[1] (0.92)	4.9[1] (0.99)	19.17[1] (0.17)

Groups with common superscript differ; $P<.05$.
[a] Adjusted for age, race, gender, baseline BMI, parent BMI, PCP age, and practice effects (clustering).
[b] Subtracting year 2 BMI percentile from baseline BMI percentile.

Secondary Outcomes

Parent self-reported fruit and vegetable intake of the index child was significantly higher in group 3 than group 1. See **Table 4**. Hours of screen time were significantly lower in group 3 compared with both group 2 and group 1. Values for physical activity and sweetened beverages generally favored group 3 but the differences were not significant.

Parents self-reported grade for their family's target behaviors are reported in **Table 5**. For all behaviors, the odds of parents reporting an A grade were higher for group 3 than group 1 and were statistically greater than 1.0 for fruit intake and physical activity. Odds of an A grade were higher in group 2 than group 1 for all but physical activity and screen time, but they were not statistically different than 1.0.

PROCESS EVALUATION OF THE BRIEF MOTIVATIONAL INTERVIEWING TO REDUCE BODY MASS INDEX
Parent Survey Data

At the end of the BMI^2, surveys were collected from 280 parents (125 from group 2 and 155 from group 3, the 2 groups that received the MI intervention). Both closed and open questions were asked about various aspects of their study experience. Overall satisfaction with the program was high, with 80% answering somewhat/very satisfied with their experience. In terms of rating the PCP and RD counseling, as shown in **Table 6**, responses were generally positive, although somewhat more so about the MD than RD counseling.

Table 3
Year 2 adjusted body mass index percentile change by motivational interview dose received—Brief Motivational Interviewing to Reduce Body Mass Index

Study Group	N	Mean Body Mass Index Percentile Change[a] (SE)
Group 1	149	1.7[1,2] (0.94)
Group 2 PCP only; low <3 MI	23	3.2 (2.1)
Group 2 PCP only; high ≥3 MI	112	4.2 (1.0)
Group 3 PCP + RD; low <8 MI	104	4.6[2] (1.0)
Group 3 PCP + RD; high ≥8 MI	37	5.5[1] (1.6)

Groups with common superscript significantly differ; $P<.05$.
[a] Adjusted for age, race, gender, baseline BMI, parent gender, household income, parent BMI, and practice effects (clustering).

Table 4
Year 2 adjusted behavioral outcomes[a]

Study Group	Fruit and Vegetables, Serving per Day (SE)	Physical Activity, Hours per Day (SE)	Sweetened Beverages, Serving per Day (SE)	Screen Time, Hours per Day (SE)
Group 1	3.8[1] (0.12)	2.1 (0.05)	1.3 (0.11)	2.5[1] (0.10)
Group 2	4.1 (0.14)	1.9 0(.06)	1.3 (0.11)	2.4[2] (0.11)
Group 3	4.3[1] (0.13)	2.1 (0.06)	1.0 (0.12)	2.2[1,2] (0.10)

Groups with common superscript significantly differ; P<.05.
[a] Adjusted means for age, race, gender, baseline value, and practice effects (clustering).

Parent Open-Ended Response

Key findings from open-ended items included a desire for more flexible times to participate in the RD phone counseling as well as a request for booster messages, ideally electronic (either SMS or e-mailed).

Registered Dietitian Interviews

All study RDs were contacted to complete a semistructured interviews focusing on elucidating the low MI completion rates in group 3. Responses were obtained from 7 (of 13 study completers) RDs. Key issues we identified were (1) providing parents with more evening and weekend hours to receive the RD counseling; (2) improving data sharing between RDs and PCPs, perhaps using a shared electronic record; (3) improving call tracking for the RDs; and (4) improving PCP endorsement of the RD counseling component.

Primary Care Provider Interviews

Seven of the 10 usual care PCPs were interviewed at their poststudy MI training, in part to elucidate the larger than expected BMI changes in the usual care group. There were not sufficient resources to interview groups 2 and 3 PCPs. Among usual care PCPs, 1 practice added an RD to their staff during the trial and 1 noted that their patients were motivated to lose weight "to make their doctor look good."

DISCUSSION AND FUTURE ENHANCEMENTS TO THE BRIEF MOTIVATIONAL INTERVIEWING TO REDUCE BODY MASS INDEX

The BMI^2 intervention achieved statistically significant and clinically meaningful[85–87] reductions in BMI percentile between groups 3 and 1 and borderline significant effects

Table 5
Odds of a parental-reported A grade[a] at 2-year follow-up for target health behaviors

Study Group	Fruits Intake	Vegetable Intake	Physical Activity	Sweetened Beverages	Eating Out	Screen Time	TV Time	Snacks
Group 1	1.0	1.0	1.0	1.0	1.0	1.0	1.0	1.0
Group 2	1.7	1.1	0.71	1.2	1.1	0.86	1.1	1.3
Group 3	2.1[1]	1.7	2.0[1]	1.4	1.8	1.4	1.8	1.7

Superscript indicates odds of parent reporting an A grade versus other grade are significantly greater than group 1.
[a] Adjusted for age, race, gender, baseline value, and practice effects (clustering).

Table 6
Parent process data collected at end of Brief Motivational Interviewing to Reduce Body Mass Index trial (n = 280)

Survey Item	Not at all (%)	A Little/ Somewhat (%)	A Lot (%)
The *doctor* asked my opinion about things.	1	24	75
The *RD* asked my opinion about things.	5	39	56
The *doctor* gave me choices about what to do.	0	22	78
The *RD* gave me choices about what to do.	5	35	60
The *doctor* listened to me.	1	6	93
The *RD* listened to me.	3	21	76
The *doctor* rushed me through the interview.	92	5	3
The *RD* rushed me through the interview.	88	7	5
The *doctor* was supportive and encouraging.	1	8	91
The *RD* was supportive and encouraging.	5	19	76
The *doctor* and I discussed values that are important to me.	0	21	79
The *RD* and I discussed values that are important to me.	6	28	66

between groups 2 and 1. These effects are, to the authors' knowledge, the largest reported for a PC intervention.[12,17,22–27] One reason for the lack of effects between groups 1 and 2 was the larger than expected change in the usual care group. Additional discussion of this issue can be found elsewhere.[19] Although the results were promising, the effects observed may have been attenuated by the lower than expected intervention dose by the group 3 RDs. Even stronger intervention effects were observed for the subset of families who completed the RD intervention. The process analyses identified several potential means to enhance intervention uptake and thereby its efficacy. Four suggestions are discussed for improving the BMI^2 model: (1) adding text messaging, (2) moving the RD counseling to a centralized disease management (DM) system, (3) integrating BMI^2 into electronic health records, and (4) providing practitioners with real-time feedback regarding their counseling via a natural language processing (NLP) system.

Text Messaging to Boost Intervention Effects, Enhance Engagement, and Reduce Attrition

One means to enhance impact and uptake of the BMI^2 intervention recommended by parents and practitioners was to add supplemental text messaging. SMS and related e-health interventions have increasingly been used to improve adherence to appointments and to deliver motivational and behavior change messages.[88–113] For BMI^2, SMS could be used to provide reminders to schedule and complete MI calls as well as deliver behavioral and motivational messages, such as goal attainment and reminders of the reasons parents and youth would benefit from controlling their weight. SMS can also be used to help track goal attainment and self-monitoring behavior changes.

Move Registered Dietitian Counseling to a Centralized Telephonic Disease Management System

A major limitation of BMI^2 was the low rate of call completion by the RDs who were linked to each PC practice. One means to improve the uptake of the RD counseling is to move this intervention component to a centralized DM system. Increasingly,

DM programs are conducted telephonically.[114–119] Telephone DM counseling has been used to address a wide range of health issues, including medication adherence,[120,121] diabetes control,[122–126] heart failure,[119,121,127] smoking cessation,[128] and adult weight management.[129–135] Many health care delivery systems, including the Department of Veterans Affairs,[125,130,136] integrative health care delivery systems,[128,137,138] and both Medicare and Medicaid,[120–123,139] use DM to manage chronic disease, and this approach seems increasingly used across the health care delivery system.[138,139] Few pediatric obesity studies have included telephone components.[23,140] Most have relied on practice staff to deliver the intervention rather than professionally trained and centrally supervised personnel. In 1 prior study as well as the BMI^2 study, parent satisfaction did not differ when delivered face to face or by telephone.[141] Also, telephonic DM programs seem more cost effective for than in-person counseling.[125,129,136,142] Advantages of a centralized DM system include (1) use of dedicated, highly trained RDs who are supervised centrally, (2) lower per-session costs than with in-person office-based interventions, and (3) greater scheduling flexibility for patients and thereby greater appointment adherence.

Integration of the Brief Motivational Interviewing to Reduce Body Mass Index into Electronic Health Records

The electronic health record offers several potential opportunities to enhance the impact of the BMI^2 and similar interventions. Prompts can be provided to remind physicians to engage parents of children with elevated BMI (BMI is typically included in most electronic health records already). Modules can be added that provide clinicians with tips (sample questions and reflections, 0–10 scales, and values lists) for using MI as well as checklists to document what was discussed during the encounter. In addition, intervention materials (eg, behavioral tips and self-monitoring tools) for parents can be incorporated into the electronic health record and sent to patients via a patient portal or other distribution mechanisms. A recent study by Taveras and colleagues[20] demonstrates the potential benefit of such systems-level interventions.

Natural Language Processing to Automatically Code Clinician Responses

At the end of the 1.5 day training for BMI^2, all clinicians completed a standardized patient session and they were provided immediate feedback about their skills. There was not the ability, however, to provide ongoing monitoring and supervision of clinicians throughout the study. In part, this was due to the effort, cost, and logistics required to provide human feedback to the clinicians. A potential solution to address this problem is to provide feedback through an automated computer system designed to perform real-time rating of clinician behaviors and summarize relevant aspects of the patient-counselor interaction. This can be accomplished through NLP. NLP is a discipline that applies computational models to understand and process text and speech data. This article reports on a preliminary proof-of-concept study using NLP to code responses by MI counselors and then compares these to code from human raters using the Motivational Interviewing Treatment Integrity (MITI) 4.0 rating system. A few prior studies have examined computer-based techniques for analyzing MI encounters.[143,144]

This pilot study focused on using NLP analyses of linguistic patterns to code 2 core MI responses: reflections and questions. The research was completed in 3 steps. First, a data set of MI encounters coded with the MITI 4.0 system was built. Second, NLP methods were used to extract and analyze linguistic patterns associated with responses coded as reflections and questions by the MITI raters. Third, an automatic system able to predict behavior codes and evaluate MI interventions was developed.

Methods

The data set is based on 284 audio recordings of MI counseling encounters from various sources, including counseling sessions from clinical trials for smoking cessation and medical adherence, students' counseling sessions from a graduate-level MI course, telephone health coaching calls, and demonstrations of MI strategies in brief medical encounters. The data set consists of a total of 97.8 hours of audio recordings with an average session duration of 20.8 minutes. Each session was transcribed and annotated by 1 of 3 coders using the MITI coding system. During the transcription process, some sessions were excluded due to recording errors, leaving 277 sessions, which were randomly distributed among the 3 coders. The annotation was conducted at utterance level by manually selecting and labeling the utterance for the specific MI behavior present in that utterance.

Once the annotation was completed, the data were processed to extract the verbal content. The final set contains 15,886 counseling behavior annotations distributed among 10 MITI codes as follows: 5262 questions, 2690 simple reflections, 2876 complex reflections, 614 seeking collaboration, 141 emphasizing autonomy, 499 affirm, 141 confront, 598 persuading without permission, 1017 giving information, and 2100 persuading with permission. This article reports results only for reflections (combining complex and simple) and questions.

Reliability of the Human Coders

Coding reliability was measured in a sample of 10 double-coded sessions, which contained a total of 546 annotations. To compare annotations for each MI behavior, all the annotations from each coder were extracted and paired at utterance level. Because the coding was performed without previous preparsing, parsing differences were addressed by applying utterance-matching methods that dealt with differences in utterance boundaries and with utterances split among 2 codes. An annotation match was assigned when both coders agreed on their evaluations. Utterances for which a matching pair was unable to be found or that differed on the assigned codes were regarded as disagreements. For this pilot study, the coders' reliability for reflections and questions was measured, and the intraclass correlation coefficient was measured at 0.97, 0.82, and 0.89 for questions, simple reflections, and complex reflections, respectively. Their pairwise agreements using Cohen's kappa metric, which accounts for the probability of agreement by chance, were 0.64, 0.34, and 0.39, for questions, simple reflections, and complex reflections, respectively.

Statistical Classification of Motivational Interviewing Behaviors

To explore the linguistic patterns for reflections and questions, the verbal content of the samples for each behavior using the following linguistic features was analyzed.

N-grams

N-grams represent the language used by the counselor and include all the unique words and word pairs present in counselor speech while making reflective statements or questions. For instance, words and word pairs, such as *sounds, like, feeling, change, to, sounds-like, feeling-like,* and *to-change,* form part of the reflections language. To obtain these features, a vocabulary was first built containing all the unique words from all the behavior annotations and then the frequency of each unique word and word pair in each annotation was counted. Thus, a vector containing the frequencies of each word and word pair in the annotation was obtained.

Semantic information

Semantic features attempt to bring semantic meaning into the analysis of counselor language by identifying words belonging to specific semantic categories, for instance, tentative language: *maybe, perhaps, guess,* and *looks,* and anxiety words: *afraid, tense,* and *worried.* Two different groups of semantic features were used. The first consists of features derived from the Linguistic Inquiry and Word Count lexicon,[142] a psycholinguistic resource that contains word classes that represent psychological cues to human thought processes, emotional states, intentions, and motivations. The second is a self-acquired MI lexicon that was created by compiling a set of words frequently present during reflective statements created by the team. These features are represented as the total frequency counts of all the words in a word category that are present in counselor language.

Similarity

Because reflective listening includes repetition and rephrasing, observing linguistic similarity between client and counselor speech can be expected. Thus, the degree to which the counselor matches the client language by using linguistic style matching,[143] a computational linguistics technique that allows to quantify the extent in which 1 person use comparable types of words than the other, was measured. Linguistic style matching was measured at turn-by-turn level using the Linguistic Inquiry and Word Count word categories, for example, positive words, articles, pronouns, negations, and quantifiers. To capture information from return statements, client speech from the previous and current turn was combined along with the counselor speech corresponding to the current turn. Each of these features is represented by a score ranging between 0 and 1 that indicates the degree to which the counselor and client use the same type of words. For instance, if the feature is *anxiety,* a score close to 1 indicates the counselor and client have high degree of style matching on the use of anxiety words, which represents cases of the counselor simply repeating the same word, for example, client utterance, "I'm worried that...," and counselor utterance, "you are worried," or rephrasing with a synonym or related word, for example, "you are overwhelmed..."

Deep syntax

Deep syntax reflects the syntactic structure of the counselor statements. These features are used to encode information about the word order in the sentence. First, a sentence is represented using its dependency tree, a representation that indicates the grammatical relations between words. For instance, in the counselor utterance, "you feel sad," first each element in the sentence is assigned a speech tag: *you* (pronoun), *feel* (verb), and *sad* (adjective). Then, the relations between the words are indicated: pronoun→*you*, verb→*feel*, adjective→*sad*, nounPhrase→pronoun, verbPhrase→ verb + adjective, and sentence→nounPhrase + verbPhrase. Using this strategy, all the annotations are analyzed to find the most frequent syntactic patterns in counselor reflections and questions. The authors expect that these patterns likely capture reflection starters commonly used by the counselor, such as "it sounds like you..." Each pattern then is represented as a feature by counting how many times it occurs in the given sample.

After the feature extraction, whether these features can be used as predictors for reflections and questions using the MITI code as the reference standard is explored. Thus, a binary prediction task is performed, where annotations are classified as reflection (either simple or complex) or nonreflection (ie, statements labeled with any other MITI code). This was repeated for questions. A support vector machines[144] classifier was used, which is an algorithm that uses a set of training examples marked as belonging to 1 of 2 categories, for example, reflection and nonreflections, to build a model that learns a linear separation function that assigns new examples into 1 category or another. Several classification models are built using each of the features sets described previously. How each method was able to correctly identify reflections or questions compared with MITI codes was evaluated, using 4 standard classification measures: (1) precision, defined as the number of correctly predicted reflections or questions by the NLP compared with the MITI code for that corresponding text divided by the total number of each code predicted by NLP as reflections or questions (similar to true positives); (2) recall, which is the number of correctly identified reflections or questions by NLP compared with MITI, divided by the total number of reflections or questions identified by MITI codes; (3) F1 score, which is the harmonic mean of precision and recall; and (4) accuracy, defined as the sum of true positives and true negatives divided by the total number of all codes, that is, percentage of reflections and nonreflections (or, questions and nonquestions) correctly identified by NLP method.

In addition, each classifier was evaluated using a 5-fold cross-validation; thus, the average of 5 runs was reported, where the model was built using 80% of the data and tested on the remaining 20%. **Table 7** shows the classification results for both reflections and questions. As reference value, a majority baseline is used, which is the percentage of instances correctly classified when selecting by default the most frequent category in the training data. For instance, given that 10,320 of 15,886 training samples are nonreflections, the majority baseline for reflections is 64%. Also, because the semantic and similarity features were developed specifically for reflections, these features are not used to predict questions.

Results show that detecting reflections by automatic means yields good performance. Reflections accuracy ranged from 63% to 87% whereas questions detection accuracy ranged from 54% to 91%. Syntactic structure was a good predictor of questions and reflections as the deep syntax model shows the best tradeoff between precision and recall with F scores of 84% and 87%, respectively. Overall, these experiments support the use of automatic means to predict counselor behavior. Next steps in this research include using NLP to predict global scores, such as empathy, and building a tool to provide clinicians with real-time feedback based on the NLP analyses.

Table 7
Classification results for counselor reflections and questions using a support vector machines classifier

Feature Group	Reflections				Questions			
	Accuracy (%)	Precision (%)	Recall (%)	F Score (%)	Accuracy (%)	Precision (%)	Recall (%)	F Score (%)
Baseline	64	0	0	0	66	0	0	0
N-grams	83	78	80	79	54	38	35	36
Semantic information	72	67	51	58	NA	NA	NA	NA
Similarity	63	58	27	37	NA	NA	NA	NA
Deep syntax	87	82	86	84	91	90	88	87

CLOSING

In addition to the issues discussed previously, bringing the BMI^2 intervention to scale will also require addressing other key challenges, including (1) how to deliver the MI training component across large health systems, perhaps using Web-based or tele-health strategies; (2) maximizing reimbursement for providers from both government and private payers; and (3) adapting the intervention to current policy changes and the evolving health care delivery system, such as requirements set forth in the Afford-able Care Act.

ACKNOWLEDGMENTS

We thank the 41 PROS practitioners, their office staffs, and the registered dietitians of the Dietetics Practice-Based Research Network for their participation. We also acknowledge the many contributions of Eric J. Slora, PhD, and Alison Bocian, MS, to the design and implementation of the study.

REFERENCES

1. Skinner A, Skelton JA. PRevalence and trends in obesity and severe obesity among children in the united states, 1999-2012. JAMA Pediatr 2014;168(6):561–6.
2. Ogden CL, Carroll MD, Kit BK, et al. PRevalence of childhood and adult obesity in the united states, 2011-2012. JAMA 2014;311(8):806–14.
3. Lee WW. An overview of pediatric obesity. Pediatr Diabetes 2007;8(Suppl 9): 76–87.
4. Finkelstein E, Fiebelkorn I, Wang G. National medical spending attributable to over-weight and obesity: how much, and who's paying? Health Aff 2003;W3:219–26.
5. Wolf A, Colditz GA. Current estimates of the economic cost of obesity in the United States. Obes Res 1998;6(2):97–106.
6. Must A, Spadano J, Coakley EH, et al. the disease burden associated with over-weight and obesity. JAMA 1999;282(16):1523–9.
7. Dietz W. Health consequences of obesity in youth: childhood predictors of adult disease. Pediatrics 1998;101(Suppl 3):518–25.
8. Mayfield CA, Suminski RR. Addressing obesity with pediatric patients and their families in a primary care office. Prim Care 2015;42(1):151–7.
9. Klein JD, Sesselberg TS, Johnson MS, et al. Adoption of body mass index guidelines for screening and counseling in pediatric practice. Pediatrics 2010; 125(2):265–72.
10. Epstein LH, Paluch RA, Roemmich JN, et al. Family-based obesity treatment, then and now: twenty-five years of pediatric obesity treatment. Health Psychol 2007;26(4):381–91.
11. Magarey AM, Perry RA, Baur LA, et al. A parent-led family-focused treatment program for overweight children aged 5 to 9 years: the PEACH RCT. Pediatrics 2011;127(2):214–22.
12. Nowicka P, Flodmark CE. Family in pediatric obesity management: a literature review. Int J Pediatr Obes 2008;3(Suppl 1):44–50.
13. Kalarchian MA, Levine MD, Arslanian SA, et al. Family-based treatment of severe pediatric obesity: randomized, controlled trial. Pediatrics 2009;124(4): 1060–8.
14. Resnicow K, Yaroch A, Davis A, et al. GO GIRLS!: results from a pilot nutrition and physical activity program for low-income overweight African American adolescent females. Health Educ Behav 2000;27(5):633–48.

15. Resnicow K, Taylor R, Baskin M. Results of go girls: a nutrition and physical activity intervention for overweight African American adolescent females conducted through Black churches. Obes Res 2005;13(10):1739–48.
16. Epstein LH, Paluch RA, Beecher MD, et al. Increasing healthy eating vs. reducing high energy-dense foods to treat pediatric obesity. Obesity (Silver Spring) 2008; 16(2):318–26.
17. Schwartz RP, Hamre R, Dietz WH, et al. Office-based motivational interviewing to prevent childhood obesity: a feasibility study. Arch Pediatr Adolesc Med 2007;161(5):495–501.
18. Resnicow K, McMaster F, Woolford S, et al. Study design and baseline description of the BMI2 trial: reducing paediatric obesity in primary care practices. Pediatr Obes 2012;7(1):3–15.
19. Resnicow K, McMaster F, Bocian A, et al. Motivational Interviewing and dietary counseling for obesity in primary care: an RCT. Pediatrics 2015;135(4):649–57.
20. Taveras EM, Marshall R, Kleinman KP, et al. Comparative effectiveness of childhood obesity interventions in pediatric primary care: a cluster-randomized clinical trial. JAMA Pediatr 2015;169(6):535–42.
21. Pakpour AH, Gellert P, Dombrowski SU, et al. Motivational interviewing with parents for obesity: an RCT. Pediatrics 2015;135(3):e644–52.
22. Whitlock EP, O'Connor EA, Williams SB, et al. Effectiveness of weight management interventions in children: a targeted systematic review for the USPSTF. Pediatrics 2010;125(2):e396–418.
23. Taveras EM, Gortmaker SL, Hohman KH, et al. Randomized controlled trial to improve primary care to prevent and manage childhood obesity: the high five for kids study. Arch Pediatr Adolesc Med 2011;165(8):714–22.
24. Taveras EM, Hohman KH, Price SN, et al. Correlates of participation in a pediatric primary care-based obesity prevention intervention. Obesity (Silver Spring) 2011;19(2):449–52.
25. Saelens BE, Sallis JF, Wilfley DE, et al. Behavioral weight control for overweight adolescents initiated in primary care. Obes Res 2002;10(1):22–32.
26. Kelishadi R, Malekahmadi M, Hashemipour M, et al. Can a trial of motivational lifestyle counseling be effective for controlling childhood obesity and the associated cardiometabolic risk factors? Pediatr Neonatal 2012;53(2):90–7.
27. McCallum Z, Wake M, Gerner B, et al. Outcome data from the LEAP (Live, Eat and Play) trial: a randomized controlled trial of a primary care intervention for childhood overweight/mild obesity. Int J Obes (Lond) 2007;31(4):630–6.
28. Norman G, Huang J, Davila EP, et al. Outcomes of a 1-year randomized controlled trial to evaluate a behavioral 'stepped-down' weight loss intervention for adolescent patients with obesity. Pediatr Obes 2016;11(1):18–25.
29. Story MT, Neumark-Stzainer DR, Sherwood NE, et al. Management of child and adolescent obesity: attitudes, barriers, skills, and training needs among health care professionals. Pediatrics 2002;110(1):210–4.
30. Brown J, Weedn A, Gillaspy S. Childhood obesity management in primary care: a needs assessment of pediatricians to guide resource development. J Okla State Med Assoc 2014;107(9–10):518–22.
31. Rausch JC, Rothbaum Perito E, Hametz P. Obesity prevention, screening, and treatment: practices of pediatric providers since the 2007 Expert Committee Recommendations. Clin Pediatr 2011;50(5):434–41.
32. Moyce SC, Bell JF. Receipt of pediatric weight-related counseling and screening in a national sample after the Expert Committee Recommendations. Clin Pediatr (Phila) 2015;54(14):1366–74.

33. Jelalian E, Boergers J, Alday CS, et al. Survey of physician attitudes and practices related to pediatric obesity. Clin Pediatr 2003;42(3):235–45.

34. Davis MM, Gance-Cleveland B, Hassink S, et al. Recommendations for Prevention of Childhood Obesity. Pediatrics 2007;120(Suppl 4):S229–53.

35. Spear BA, Barlow SE, Ervin C, et al. Recommendations for treatment of child and adolescent overweight and obesity. Pediatrics 2007;120(Suppl 4):S254–88.

36. Resnicow K, Davis R, Rollnick S. Motivational interviewing for pediatric obesity: conceptual issues and evidence review. J Am Diet Assoc 2006;106(12): 2024–33.

37. Flattum C, Friend S, Neumark-Sztainer D, et al. Motivational interviewing as a component of a school-based obesity prevention program for adolescent girls. J Am Diet Assoc 2009;109(1):91–4.

38. Brennan L, Walkley J, Fraser SF, et al. Motivational interviewing and cognitive behaviour therapy in the treatment of adolescent overweight and obesity: study design and methodology. Contemp Clin Trials 2008;29(3):359–75.

39. Carels RA, Darby L, Cacciapaglia HM, et al. Using motivational interviewing as a supplement to obesity treatment: a stepped-care approach. Health Psychol 2007;26(3):369–74.

40. Irby M, Kaplan S, Garner-Edwards D, et al. Motivational interviewing in a family-based pediatric obesity program: a case study. Fam Syst Health 2010;28(3): 236–46.

41. MacDonell K, Brogan K, Naar-King S, et al. A pilot study of motivational interviewing targeting weight-related behaviors in overweight or obese African American Adolescents. J Adolesc Health 2012;50(2):201–3.

42. Resnicow K, McMaster F. Motivational interviewing: moving from why to how with autonomy support. Int J Behav Nutr Phys Act 2012;9:19.

43. Resnicow K, McMaster F, Rollnick S. Action Reflections: a client-centered technique to bridge the WHY-HOW transition in motivational interviewing. Behav Cognit Psychother 2012;40(4):474–80.

44. Bem D. Self-perception theory. In: Berkowitz L, editor. Advances in experimetnal social psychology, vol. 6. New York: Academic Press; 1972. p. 1–62.

45. Resnicow K, Gobat N, Naar S. Intensifying and igniting change talk in Motivational Interviewing: a theoretical and practical framework. European Health Psychologist 2015;17(3):102–10.

46. Barnett E, Moyers TB, Sussman S, et al. From counselor skill to decreased marijuana use: does change talk matter? J Subst Abuse Treat 2014;46(4):498–505.

47. Gaume J, Bertholet N, Faouzi M, et al. Does change talk during brief motivational interventions with young men predict change in alcohol use? J Subst Abuse Treat 2013;44(2):177–85.

48. Glynn LH, Moyers TB. Chasing change talk: the clinician's role in evoking client language about change. J Subst Abuse Treat 2010;39(1):65–70.

49. Moyers TB, Martin T, Houck JM, et al. From in-session behaviors to drinking outcomes: a causal chain for motivational interviewing. J Consult Clin Psychol 2009;77(6):1113–24.

50. Miller WR, Rose GS. Toward a theory of motivational interviewing. Am Psychol 2009;64(6):527–37.

51. Miller WR, Rollnick S. Motivational interviewing: help people change. 3rd edition. New York: Guilford Press; 2013.

52. Gaume J, McCambridge J, Bertholet N, et al. Mechanisms of action of brief alcohol interventions remain largely unknown – a narrative review. Front Psychiatry 2014;5:108.

53. Magill M, Gaume J, Apodaca TR, et al. The technical hypothesis of motivational interviewing: a meta-analysis of MI's key causal model. J Consult Clin Psychol 2014;82(6):973–83.

54. Vader AM, Walters ST, Prabhu GC, et al. The language of motivational interviewing and feedback: counselor language, client language, and client drinking outcomes. Psychol Addict Behav 2010;24(2):190–7.

55. Amrhein PC, Miller WR, Yahne CE, et al. Client commitment language during motivational interviewing predicts drug use outcomes. J Consult Clin Psychol 2003;71(5):862–78.

56. Carcone AI, Naar-King S, Brogan KE, et al. Provider communication behaviors that predict motivation to change in black adolescents with obesity. J Dev Behav Pediatr 2013;34(8):599–608.

57. Barlow SE. Expert committee recommendations regarding the prevention, assessment, and treatment of child and adolescent overweight and obesity: summary report. Pediatrics 2007;120(Suppl 4):S164–92.

58. Centers for Disease Control. BMI calculator. 2011. Available at: https://nccd.cdc.gov/dnpabmi/calculator.aspx. Accessed March 03, 2016.

59. Wasserman RC, Croft CA, Brotherton SE. Preschool vision screening in pediatric practice: a study from the Pediatric Research in Office Settings (PROS) Network. American Academy of Pediatrics. Pediatrics 1992; 89(5 Pt 1):834–8.

60. Kelleher KJ. Insurance status and recognition of psychosocial problems. A report from the Pediatric Research in Office Settings and the Ambulatory Sentinel Practice Networks. Arch Pediatr Adolesc Med 1997;151(11):1109–15.

61. Forrest CB, Glade GB, Baker AE, et al. The pediatric primary-specialty care interface: how pediatricians refer children and adolescents to specialty care. Arch Pediatr Adolesc Med 1999;153(7):705–14.

62. Slora EJ, Thoma KA, Wasserman RC, et al. Patient visits to a national practice-based research network: comparing pediatric research in office settings with the National Ambulatory Medical Care Survey. Pediatrics 2006;118(2):e228–34.

63. Rollnick S, Butler CC, Stott N. Helping smokers make decisions: the enhancement of brief intervention for general medical practice. Patient Educ Couns 1997;31(3):191–203.

64. Rollnick S, Heather N, Gold R, et al. Development of a short "readiness to change" questionnaire for use in brief, opportunistic interventions among excessive drinkers. Br J Addict 1992;87(5):743–54.

65. Rollnick S, Mason P, Butler C. Health behavior change: a guide for practitioners. London: Churchill Livingstone (Harcourt Brace Inc); 1999.

66. Rollnick S, Butler C, Cambridge J, et al. Consultations about behaviour change. BMJ 2005;331(7522):961–3.

67. Rollnick S, Miller W, Butler C. Motivational interviewing in health care: helping patients change behavior. New York: Guilford Publications; 2007.

68. Emmons K, Rollnick S. Motivational interviewing in health care settings: opportunities and limitations. Am J Prev Med 2001;20(1):68–74.

69. Resnicow K, DiIorio C, Soet J, et al. Motivational interviewing in medical and public health settings. In: Miller W, Rollnick S, editors. Motivational interviewing: preparing people for change. 2nd edition. New York: Guildford Press; 2002. p. 251–69.

70. Resnicow K, DiIorio C, Soet JE, et al. Motivational interviewing in health promotion: it sounds like something is changing. Health Psychol 2002;21(5):444–51.

71. Rollnick S, Allison J, Ballasiotes S, et al. Variations on a theme: motivational interviewing and its adaptations. In: Miller W, Rollnick S, editors. Motivational interviewing. 2nd edition. New York: Guildford Publications Inc; 2002. p. 270–83.

72. Butler C, Rollnick S, Cohen D, et al. Motivational consulting versus brief advice for smokers in general practice: a randomized trial. Br J Gen Pract 1999;49: 611–6.

73. Butler CC, Pill R, Stott NC. Qualitative study of patients' perceptions of doctors' advice to quit smoking: implications for opportunistic health promotion. BMJ 1998;316:1878–81.

74. Butler CC, Rollnick S, Pill R, et al. Understanding the culture of prescribing: qualitative study of general practitioners' and patients' perceptions of antibiotics for sore throats. BMJ 1998;317(7159):637–42.

75. Stott NCH, Rollnick S, Pill RM. Innovation in clinical method: diabetes care and negotiating skills. Fam Pract 1995;12(4):413–8.

76. Miller W, Mount K. A small study of training in motivational interviewing: does one workshop change clinician and client behavior? Behav Cognit Psychother 2001;29:457–71.

77. Velasquez M, Hecht J, Quinn V, et al. Application of motivational interviewing to prenatal smoking cessation: training and implementation issues. Tob Control 2000;9(Suppl 3):III36–40.

78. McMaster F, Resnicow K. Validation of the one pass measure for motivational interviewing competence. Patient Educ Couns 2015;98(4):499–505.

79. Flynn MA, McNeil DA, Maloff B, et al. Reducing obesity and related chronic disease risk in children and youth: a synthesis of evidence with 'best practice' recommendations. Obes Rev 2006;7(Suppl 1):7–66.

80. Ludwig DS, Peterson KE, Gortmaker SL. Relation between consumption of sugar-sweetened drinks and childhood obesity: a prospective, observational analysis. Lancet 2001;357(9255):505–8.

81. Bray GA, Nielsen SJ, Popkin BM. Consumption of high-fructose corn syrup in beverages may play a role in the epidemic of obesity. Am J Clin Nutr 2004; 79(4):537–43.

82. Evidence Library. Available at: http://www.adaevidencelibrary.org/. Accessed March 03, 2016.

83. Vansteenkiste M, Williams GC, Resnicow K. Toward systematic integration between self-determination theory and motivational interviewing as examples of top-down and bottom-up intervention development: autonomy or volition as a fundamental theoretical principle. Int J Behav Nutr Phys Act 2012;9:23.

84. Murray D. Design and analysis of group randomized trials, vol. 27. New York: Oxford University Press; 1998.

85. Frohlich G, Pott W, Albayrak O, et al. Conditions of long-term success in a lifestyle intervention for overweight and obese youths. Pediatrics 2011;128(4): e779–85.

86. Reinehr T, Kiess W, Kapellen T, et al. to Degree of Weight Loss. Pediatrics 2004; 114(6):1569–73.

87. Ford AL, Hunt LP, Cooper A, et al. What reduction in BMI SDS is required in obese adolescents to improve body composition and cardiometabolic health? Arch Dis Child 2010;95(4):256–61.

88. Hurling R, Catt M, De Boni M, et al. Using internet and mobile phone technology to deliver an automated physical activity program: randomized controlled Trial. J Med Internet Res 2007;9(2):e7.

89. Corrigan MA, McHugh SM, Murphy RK, et al. Improving surgical outpatient efficiency through mobile phone text messaging. Surg Innov 2011;18(4):354–7.

90. Kachur R, Adelson S, Firenze K, et al. Reaching patients and their partners through mobile: text messaging for case management and partner notification. Sex Transm Dis 2011;38(2):149–50.

91. Wei J, Hollin I, Kachnowski S. A review of the use of mobile phone text messaging in clinical and healthy behaviour interventions. J Telemed Telecare 2011;17(1):41–8.

92. Prabhakaran L, Chee WY, Chua KC, et al. The use of text messaging to improve asthma control: a pilot study using the mobile phone short messaging service (SMS). J Telemed Telecare 2010;16(5):286–90.

93. Shapiro JR, Bauer S, Andrews E, et al. Mobile therapy: Use of text-messaging in the treatment of bulimia nervosa. Int J Eat Disord 2010;43(6):513–9.

94. Gerber BS, Stolley MR, Thompson AL, et al. Mobile phone text messaging to promote healthy behaviors and weight loss maintenance: a feasibility study. Health Informatics J 2009;15(1):17–25.

95. Mao Y, Zhang Y, Zhai S. Mobile phone text messaging for pharmaceutical care in a hospital in China. J Telemed Telecare 2008;14(8):410–4.

96. Riley W, Obermayer J, Jean-Mary J. Internet and mobile phone text messaging intervention for college smokers. J Am Coll Health 2008;57(2):245–8.

97. Lim MS, Hocking JS, Hellard ME, et al. SMS STI: a review of the uses of mobile phone text messaging in sexual health. Int J STD AIDS 2008;19(5):287–90.

98. Wangberg SC, Arsand E, Andersson N. Diabetes education via mobile text messaging. J Telemed Telecare 2006;12(Suppl 1):55–6.

99. Rodgers A, Corbett T, Bramley D, et al. Do u smoke after txt? Results of a randomised trial of smoking cessation using mobile phone text messaging. Tob Control 2005;14(4):255–61.

100. Yoong JK. Mobile phones can be a pain–text messaging tenosynovitis. Hosp Med 2005;66(6):370.

101. Bramley D, Riddell T, Whittaker R, et al. Smoking cessation using mobile phone text messaging is as effective in Maori as non-Maori. N Z Med J 2005;118(1216):U1494.

102. Ferrer-Roca O, Cardenas A, Diaz-Cardama A, et al. Mobile phone text messaging in the management of diabetes. J Telemed Telecare 2004;10(5):282–5.

103. Neville R, Greene A, McLeod J, et al. Mobile phone text messaging can help young people manage asthma. BMJ 2002;325(7364):600.

104. Burke LE, Conroy MB, Sereika SM, et al. The effect of electronic self-monitoring on weight loss and dietary intake: a randomized behavioral weight loss trial. Obesity (Silver Spring) 2011;19(2):338–44.

105. Free C, Phillips G, Watson L, et al. The effectiveness of mobile-health technologies to improve health care service delivery processes: a systematic review and meta-analysis. PLoS Med 2013;10(1):e1001363.

106. Car J, Ng C, Atun R, et al. SMS text message healthcare appointment reminders in England. J Ambul Care Manage 2008;31(3):216–9.

107. Mohammed S, Siddiqi O, Ali O, et al. User engagement with and attitudes towards an interactive SMS reminder system for patients with tuberculosis. J Telemed Telecare 2012;18(7):404–8.

108. Strandbygaard U, Thomsen SF, Backer V. A daily SMS reminder increases adherence to asthma treatment: a three-month follow-up study. Respir Med 2010;104(2):166–71.

109. Hanauer DA, Wentzell K, Laffel N, et al. Computerized Automated Reminder Diabetes System (CARDS): e-mail and SMS cell phone text messaging reminders to support diabetes management. Diabetes Technol Ther 2009;11(2): 99–106.

110. Khokhar A. Short text messages (SMS) as a reminder system for making working women from Delhi Breast Aware. Asian Pac J Cancer Prev 2009;10(2): 319–22.

111. Foley J, O'Neill M. Use of mobile telephone short message service (SMS) as a reminder: the effect on patient attendance. Eur Arch Paediatr Dent 2009; 10(1):15–8.

112. Chen ZW, Fang LZ, Chen LY, et al. Comparison of an SMS text messaging and phone reminder to improve attendance at a health promotion center: a randomized controlled trial. J Zhejiang Univ Sci B 2008;9(1):34–8.

113. Junod Perron N, Dao MD, Righini NC, et al. Text-messaging versus telephone reminders to reduce missed appointments in an academic primary care clinic: a randomized controlled trial. BMC Health Serv Res 2013;13(1):125.

114. Ellerbeck EF, Mahnken JD, Cupertino AP, et al. Effect of varying levels of disease management on smoking cessation: a randomized trial. Ann Intern Med 2009; 150(7):437–46.

115. Cupertino AP, Mahnken JD, Richter K, et al. Long-term engagement in smoking cessation counseling among rural smokers. J Health Care Poor Underserved 2007;18(Suppl 4):39–51.

116. Resnicow K, Jackson A, Braithwaite R, et al. Healthy body/healthy spirit: design and evaluation of a church-based nutrition and physical activity intervention using motivational interviewing. Health Educ Res 2002;17(2):562–73.

117. Resnicow K, Baskin M, Rahotep S, et al. Motivational interviewing in health promotion & behavioral medicine settings. In: Cox W, Klinger E, editors. Handbook of motivational counseling: motivating people for change. Sussex (United Kingdom): John Wiley and Sons; 2003. p. 457–79.

118. Resnicow K, Jackson A, Wang T, et al. A motivational interviewing intervention to increase fruit and vegetable intake through Black churches: results of the Eat for Life trial. Am J Public Health 2001;91(10):1686–93.

119. Bashshur RL, Shannon GW, Smith BR, et al. The empirical foundations of telemedicine interventions for chronic disease management. Telemed J E Health 2014;20(9):769–800.

120. Moczygemba LR, Barner JC, Gabrillo ER, et al. Development and implementation of a telephone medication therapy management program for medicare beneficiaries. Am J Health Syst Pharm 2008;65(17):1655–60.

121. Afifi AA, Morisky DE, Kominski GF, et al. Impact of disease management on health care utilization: evidence from the "Florida: A Healthy State (FAHS)" medicaid Program. Prev Med 2007;44(6):547–53.

122. Thiebaud P, Demand M, Wolf SA, et al. Impact of disease management on utilization and adherence with drugs and tests. Diabetes Care 2008;31(9): 1717–22.

123. Ratanawongsa N, Handley M, Quan J, et al. Quasi-experimental trial of diabetes Self-Management Automated and Real-Time Telephonic Support (SMARTSteps) in a medicaid managed care plan: study protocol. BMC Health Serv Res 2012; 12(1):22.

124. Berg GD, Wadhwa S. Diabetes disease management in a community-based setting. Manag Care 2002;11(6)(42):45–50.

125. Dall TM, Roary M, Yang W, et al. Health care use and costs for participants in a diabetes disease management program, United States, 2007-2008. Prev Chronic Dis 2011;8(3):A53.
126. Polisena J, Tran K, Cimon K, et al. Home telehealth for diabetes management: a systematic review and meta-analysis. Diabetes Obes Metab 2009;11(10): 913–30.
127. Clark RA, Inglis SC, McAlister FA, et al. Telemonitoring or structured telephone support programmes for patients with chronic heart failure: systematic review and meta-analysis. BMJ 2007;334(7600):942.
128. Holtrop JS, Wadland WC, Vansen S, et al. Recruiting health plan members receiving pharmacotherapy into smoking cessation counseling. Am J Manag Care 2005;11(8):501–7.
129. Digenio AG, Mancuso JP, Gerber RA, et al. Comparison of methods for delivering a lifestyle modification program for obese patients: a randomized trial. Ann Intern Med 2009;150(4):255–62.
130. Damschroder LJ, Lutes LD, Goodrich DE, et al. A small-change approach delivered via telephone promotes weight loss in veterans: Results from the ASPIRE-VA pilot study. Patient Educ Couns 2010;79(2):262–6.
131. Wilson DB, Johnson RE, Jones RM, et al. Patient weight counseling choices and outcomes following a primary care and community collaborative intervention. Patient Educ Couns 2010;79(3):338–43.
132. Sherwood NE, Jeffery RW, Welsh EM, et al. The drop it at last study: six-month results of a phone-based weight loss trial. Am J Health Promot 2010;24(6):378–83.
133. Terry PE, Seaverson ELD, Grossmeier J, et al. Effectiveness of a worksite telephone-based weight management program. Am J Health Promot 2011; 25(3):186–9.
134. Sherwood NE, Jeffery RW, Pronk NP, et al. Mail and phone interventions for weight loss in a managed-care setting: weigh-to-be 2-year outcomes. Int J Obes 2006;30(10):1565–73.
135. Sherwood NE, Crain AL, Martinson BC, et al. Keep it off: A phone-based intervention for long-term weight-loss maintenance. Contemp Clin Trials 2011;32(4): 551–60.
136. Dall TM, Askarinam Wagner RC, Zhang Y, et al. Outcomes and lessons learned from evaluating TRICARE's disease management programs. Am J Manag Care 2010;16(6):438–46.
137. Pronk NP, Boucher JL, Gehling E, et al. A platform for population-based weight management: description of a health plan-based integrated systems approach. Am J Manag Care 2002;8(10):847–57.
138. Buntin MB, Jain AK, Mattke S, et al. Who gets disease management? J Gen Intern Med 2009;24(5):649–55.
139. Goldman LE, Handley M, Rundall TG, et al. Current and future directions in medi-cal chronic disease care management: a view from the top. Am J Manag Care 2007;13(5):263–8.
140. Pinard CA, Hart MH, Hodgkins Y, et al. Smart choices for healthy families: a pilot study for the treatment of childhood obesity in low-income families. Health Educ Behav 2012;39(4):433–45.
141. Mulgrew KW, Shaikh U, Nettiksimmons J. Comparison of parent satisfaction with care for childhood obesity delivered face-to-face and by telemedicine. Telemed J E Health 2011;17(5):383–7.
142. Appel LJ, Clark JM, Yeh H-C, et al. Comparative Effectiveness of weight-loss interventions in clinical practice. N Engl J Med 2011;365(21):1959–68.

143. Lord SP, Sheng E, Imel ZE, et al. More than reflections: empathy in motivational interviewing includes language style synchrony between therapist and client. Behav Ther 2015;46(3):296–303.
144. Atkins DC, Steyvers M, Imel ZE, et al. Scaling up the evaluation of psychotherapy: evaluating motivational interviewing fidelity via statistical text classification. Implement Sci 2014;9:49.

Index

Note: Page numbers of article titles are in **boldface** type.

A

Academic performance, physical activity effects on, **459–480**
Acute bout physical activity, neurocognitive function effects of, 459–480
American Academy of Pediatrics, Pediatric Research in Office Settings network, 539–562
Autonomy, in communication, 525–538

B

Basic Behavioral and Social Science Opportunity Network, of National Institutes of Health, **389–399**
Behavioral Choice Task, 521–523
Behavioral economic factors, in obesity, **425–446**
    complementing other treatment approaches, 426, 428–440
    current state of, 440–442
    definition of, 427
    description of, 426–427
Behavioral science, for obesity interventions, **389–399**
Brief Motivational Interviewing to Reduce Body Mass Index study, 539–562

C

Cancer, obesity and, **389–399**
Cardiovascular disease, risk reduction in, 481–510
Case Western, obesity research at, 391
Change talk, 525–538
Claremont University, obesity research at, 392
Cognitive function, physical activity effects on, **459–480**
Commitment, to behavioral changes, 440
Communication, patient-provider, **525–538**
Cortisol, eating behavior and, 409–411
Counseling, patient-provider, 525–538
Cross-price elasticity, 427

D

Delay discounting, 427
Demand intensity, 427
Developmental considerations, in behavioral economics, 440
Diet, of preschoolers, 491–496
Discomfort, acceptance of, mindfulness effects on, 417

Pediatr Clin N Am 63 (2016) 563–566
http://dx.doi.org/10.1016/S0031-3955(16)30028-1
0031-3955/16/$ – see front matter

pediatric.theclinics.com

Moving?

Make sure your subscription moves with you!

To notify us of your new address, find your **Clinics Account Number** (located on your mailing label above your name), and contact customer service at:

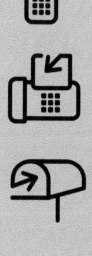

Email: journalscustomerservice-usa@elsevier.com

800-654-2452 (subscribers in the U.S. & Canada)
314-447-8871 (subscribers outside of the U.S. & Canada)

Fax number: 314-447-8029

Elsevier Health Sciences Division
Subscription Customer Service
3251 Riverport Lane
Maryland Heights, MO 63043

*To ensure uninterrupted delivery of your subscription, please notify us at least 4 weeks in advance of move.

Printed and bound by CPI Group (UK) Ltd, Croydon, CR0 4YY

08/06/2025

01896873-0011